Supporting Parent–Child Relationships From Birth

A community model for under 5s' mental health

SUSI

(Social–emotional Under 5s Screening and Intervention)

Carol Hardy and Elizabeth Murphy

Author profiles

CAROL HARDY
Carol Hardy is an under 5s Clinical Specialist and O.T. in a CAMH service in Southwark. For the past 30 years she has worked in inner city community teams and has a longstanding interest in clinical and service developments for under 5s and their birth parents, foster carers or adoptive parents. She trialled the assessment/intervention model (later known as SUSI) in a pilot project in 2010, and ran the SUSI study with Elizabeth Murphy from 2014–2017. She has developed, and delivers, consultation and training programmes on under 5s' mental health to colleagues in agencies across different settings.

ELIZABETH MURPHY
Elizabeth Murphy is a Child & Adolescent Psychotherapist and until recently was the Consultant in Carelink, the Southwark CAMHS team for Looked after and Adopted children. She has collaborated with Carol Hardy on clinical research and is interested in clinical interventions, service delivery and inter-agency work.

Acknowledgements

There are many clinical colleagues who have given energy and commitment to the babies, young children and families we have worked together with over the years and have contributed valuable insights to this work.

In the early years, the clinical practice developed through the joint work of Carol and her colleague Bernadette Kiely at Guy's Hospital. Bernadette's skill and intuitive approach to children and parents added a great deal to important learning in this clinical field. In this dedicated under 5s CAMHS team in the early 90s, supported by Tony Cox and Karin Prior, the work developed as we found new ways to engage and help the concerns families shared about their relationships with their young children.

We were later inspired by Maureen Marks to consider using clinical research to develop the ideas further. We are grateful to her, for her commitment and advice and also for facilitating the link with Susan Conroy who became the academic lead of both projects in the last 10 years in Carelink CAMHS where Carol and Elizabeth have worked. Sue's skill and steady approach guided us through complex ethical and practical processes. We are indebted to Guy's and St Thomas' Charity for funding both studies: the pilot screening project and the Social-emotional Under 4s Screening & Intervention (SUSI) study.

In both projects, clinicians and researchers have showed remarkable care and dedication to the children and parents and we are grateful to all of them. We would like to give special thanks to Elizabeth Hackett and Kate Tidnam who worked over an extended time with us.

The SUSI model has always been rooted in our local community and multi-agency context. We are indebted to a great number of colleagues in other organisations. Whilst too many to mention individually, we would like to express our appreciation of all those in Child Health, the Local Authority, and Adult/Perinatal Mental Health services along with frontline workers in Primary Care and Education. Particular people including Alasdair Smith, Helen Woolgar, April Bald, Sarah Feasey, Chris McCree and Lucy Brazener generously gave their time and insight to support the clinical work's transition to an established multiagency model.

Carol would like to thank the many people who have made significant contributions in various ways to the creation of this book with feedback, encouragement and suggestions. She is especially grateful to Carola Thorpe, Danya Glaser and Beatrice Cooper for their insights and advice. We have also greatly valued discussions and support, and been inspired by John Simmonds, Bruce Clark, Tamsin Ford, Denis Ougrin and Sarah Byford.

Finally, we would like to return to the children and families to express our appreciation of all those who over the years have participated in the clinical services or projects. Their courage to step into unknown territory at times of stress has also helped to shape our learning for this work that we hope will be of benefit to others.

Contents

Introduction

Feeling that we were supported and more importantly our child was supported and valued at such a fundamental stage of her development was appreciated by us both.

PARENTS

This under fives approach has validated my concern for the emotional well-being of babies and young children in difficult situations. It has also shown me how these problems can be assessed, understood and mitigated.

PAEDIATRICIAN

Evolution and purpose of this book

In recent decades child development research and attachment theory have highlighted the fundamental importance of the earliest relationships between parent and child, this being the 'place' where so much of a baby's mental and physical life is nurtured and developed. From a broad range of sociological and scientific work, we now have a greater awareness of the immense influence parents or primary caregivers have on their young children and how this creates huge potential for positive growth and development. This in turn creates a need and responsibility for parents and the wider family and community to support a baby's first acquaintance with the world and people around them, because the baby's experience is mediated through these caregiving relationships.

At times, these early relationships need support to help the adult caregivers manage the inherent practical and emotional demands of caring for a young infant/child. In the majority of families this 'support' is provided by a partner, the wider family and friends, with help from community healthcare and social systems. However, for a significant number of families there may be greater pressures and challenges arising from a variety of external stressors and internal unresolved trauma that mean the development of the relationship with the child is interrupted or adversely affected. This then runs the risk of impacting on the child's emotional foundation and resilience.

This handbook describes a clinical model developed in 'real world' community services. It is designed to promote and support the earliest parent–child relationships and infant mental health in a wide range of families, including those facing the greatest adversity. The model is commonly known by its acronym SUSI: Social–emotional Under 5s Screening and Intervention (Hardy & Murphy, 2018) and has been cited as an innovative practice model in a number of reports and reviews concerning infant mental health (see 'Notes' at the end of this chapter for details).

The SUSI model brings together more than 25 years of clinical work in child mental health community settings, which was articulated in a framework for recent clinical research studies (Hardy, 2001; Hardy et al., 2015; Hardy & Murphy, 2018).

We have presented the model to audiences of professionals working in a variety of settings, and have received many requests for detailed guidance on implementation. This handbook, therefore, describes how the approach was developed from both a service and research perspective. It explains how the work can be used to help parents and children, as well as implementing it within a professional team and the wider community services. This is not a manual, because the approach is tailor-made; the key principles and components, and examples of them, are described in the book.

The core approach works to highlight relational and developmental needs of a young infant/child so that their primary caregivers and wider support systems of family and/or professionals can work together to make a difference to the 'here and now' everyday experiences of the child and to fulfil their future potential. These experiences are what create our inner worlds; that is a template through which we experience subsequent relationships and events.

The early chapters focus on ideas that influenced the development of the model from everyday practice, together with evidence from the research literature. Later chapters give a more detailed breakdown of the different stages of the model including:

1. the ways in which the model can be implemented with families and partner agencies, e.g. see Chapters 2, 3 and 8.
2. the specific components in the assessment and feedback stage, e.g. see Chapter 4.
3. the techniques in the intervention stages, e.g. see Chapters 5 and 6.

As these stages were created to take an individual approach to each child and family's experience, the work is tailored to make it accessible and meaningful for everyone involved. A combination of different techniques makes this possible. The clinical work has always taken place within multi-disciplinary teams and wider multi-agency networks. Some of the challenges and solutions in relation to providing a new service are described in the later sections, with guidance for implementation in services elsewhere.

Our intention is that the book will be used by practitioners interested in promoting the emotional health and attachment needs of babies and children. It is also designed as a reference book for those wishing to undertake the training and deliver these specific clinical approaches in their current teams, or when developing new ones (see Chapter 9). As the model has defined processes and stages, it can be used by professionals who want to integrate the assessment techniques in their existing frameworks. Others may wish to implement all of the stages.

As the social, cultural and family contexts for the babies, children and parents who have taken part in both the services and research studies are so varied, we have focused on the core elements of the approach. Some sections define ways in which the work was tailored to certain populations, with generic examples from the clinical service and research studies.

Background

There is a strong body of research evidence showing that the care of prenatal, babies and young children creates a blueprint for later health and development. The 'Building Great Britons' report (2015) draws on comprehensive reviews across clinical, academic and health/social policy fields. It describes a holistic view of the wide range of health and social needs of all children in their early years, highlighting the serious impact on all aspects of development for those that face the greatest adversity and challenges. These reviews have emphasised how a child's later well-being is developed within the primary caregiving relationships, which can have more or less positive implications for the youngest in our society (The National Scientific Council on the Developing Child, 2014, NSPCC 2016). For centuries there has been a belief that influences from early childhood have long reaching effects – 'train up a child in the way he should go: and when he is old, he will not depart from it' (Proverbs, 22:6). The rapidly growing neurobiological evidence stresses how a child's earliest caregiving experience can influence all areas of their development, including at the most basic neurological level (Teicher & Samson, 2016). Infant mental health expert, Selma Fraiberg, has spoken of how 'the human capacities for love and learning are rooted in ... the first eighteen months of life' (1980).

Guidance from the National Institute for Health & Care Excellence (NICE, 2012) has highlighted gaps in the UK evidence for the effectiveness of early interventions to address social-emotional well-being of children in the early years. It has called for more evidence on the impact of such interventions on specific groups of children (minority ethnic groups and children whose parents have mental health problems).

Earlier NICE guidance for looked after children (2010) had stated that all under 5 year olds should receive a screening and timely intervention by a specialist child mental health practitioner. There is a growing acceptance of the scale of the problem, together with recognition of the consequences to the individuals and society now and in the future if we do not intervene. This is highlighted in the Early Intervention Foundation report (EIF; 2016) on the cost of 'late intervention' services provided to children experiencing difficulties later in childhood/young adulthood. The cost is estimated at £17 billion, with costs to the Local Authority of £6.4 billion, £3.7 billion for the NHS and £2.7 billion for the Department for Work and Pensions.

Along with these concerning statistics, our increased awareness and knowledge is not being translated into adequate service provision (Moriarty, Baginsky, Gorin, Baginsky & Manthorpe, 2016; NSPCC, 2016) partly due to a debate on how to target resources. The EIF report suggests that targeted interventions responding to early signs of problems in attachment security, behavioural self-regulation or early learning are more effective than universal programmes.

In general, low numbers of babies and pre-school children are being referred to and/or seen in clinical services with the expertise to identify social-emotional or mental health problems in this age range (Foreman, 2015; PIP UK, 2019). Provision of infant/child mental health assessments and interventions for this age group is patchy from providers in both public and independent services across the UK and elsewhere (NSPCC, 2016). Barger, Rice and Roach (2018) outline several key reasons why the majority of children aged 3–5 years at risk of developing these difficulties are not identified in a timely way and therefore not accessing early interventions.

These include:

- a lack of robust surveillance methods
- inadequate training of professionals across both universal and specialist services
- absence of services to refer to once a need is identified
- difficulties in the engagement of families at all stages of the process.

They conclude 'only a fraction of assessed children eligible for Early Intervention (EI) or mental health treatment ultimately receive services'.

There is extensive evidence from developmental research that different domains of a child's development influence one another and are inextricably linked. These impact on one another and affect 'progress' and expression of the child's potential. Although the mechanisms that organise pathways between physical, developmental and mental well-being remain unclear, a number of studies have demonstrated how early social-emotional adversity impacts on people at a physiological level. An example is the functioning of the hypothalamus, pituitary and adrenal (HPA) stress response system, with chronic changes to the pattern of cortisol secretion (Hertzman & Boyce, 2010), which is associated with behavioural, cognitive and emotional problems (Lomanowska, Boivin, Hertzman & Fleming, 2015). Both positive and traumatic experiences are 'remembered' in the body from the earliest everyday care, which babies are dependent on for their basic survival (Music, 2011). While there is now greater awareness and focus from research regarding the association between the emotional caregiving a child receives and their physical health, there remains a need to be alert to possible organic causes in a young child's presentation, which may be putting strain on the child-parent relationship and which need further investigation in their own right (Dabrowska & Pisula, 2010).

The infant and child

It is useful to review how current thinking informs our understanding of social-emotional development and infant mental health. One reason for carrying out the Social-emotional Under 4s Screening and Intervention (SUSI) clinical research study was to contribute to the understanding of how social-emotional and emerging mental health needs present in babies and young children in high risk or vulnerable populations.

Starting with the question of what we mean by social–emotional development and infant mental health, the National Institute for Health and Care Excellence (NICE) (2012) describes social and emotional well-being as 'providing the building block for healthy behaviours and educational attainment. It also helps prevent behavioural problems (including substance misuse) and mental illness'. It defines it as consisting of the following three components.

- **Emotional well-being** – this includes being happy and confident and not anxious or depressed.
- **Psychological well-being** – this includes the ability to be autonomous, problem-solve, manage emotions, experience empathy, and be resilient and attentive.
- **Social well-being** – has good relationships with others and does not have behavioural problems, that is, they are not disruptive, violent or a bully.

It would be difficult, inappropriate and probably unhelpful to separate out and define very young children's social–emotional presentations too concretely. This is because it may only capture one or two aspects of their difficulties and strengths at a particular time. With such rapid growth and potential for change, there is a risk that concerns remain unidentified and mislabelled and therefore remain inaccessible to support and input. This dilemma is perhaps reflected in some of the guidance and policy documents. They rightly describe the importance of the early years, identifying the components of the parenting relationship that helps to promote strong emotional foundations in the child. However, the documents provide less detail on how either positive or disturbed emotional development manifests itself in the child or within the child–parent relationship.

Reasons for this dilemma include a possible wish to avoid thoughts about the emotional impact of distress experienced by a baby or child, a period of life generally associated with joy and hope (Balbernie, 2016). It is perhaps easier to observe and define positive parenting behaviour and responses (e.g. being sensitive/responsive, setting limits) or make general reference to the child's attachment. Parents can communicate how they experience and see their child's needs, but this may not fully reflect the child's experience when too young to have a 'voice' and articulate their view.

This leads us to question how we assess the child's presentation while addressing the need recognised by experts to give consideration to the influence from the primary caregiving relationship, and the importance of the relational context (Barlow, 2015; Zeanah, Berlin & Boris, 2011; Boris, Fueyo & Zeanah, 1997).

When trying to obtain a profile of the child's social-emotional well-being and mental health, professionals need to feel sufficiently confident and clear in their view of whether the child's presentation warrants further clinical intervention. This seems to pose greater difficulties than a decision to offer a family more general social support, in the hope that this will have a beneficial impact on the child. In the absence of overt behavioural indicators of distress or difficulties that impact on others, the concerns may be often expressed in common problems that all young children experience from time to time, e.g. problem feeding or sleeping, which can be explained as within the normal range or a 'passing phase'. Added to these factors the reality is that some babies and young children show no overt signs of distress, but rather a lack of ordinary responses, e.g. do not seek comfort or attention. This may go unrecognised by the parent, particularly if they received impoverished parenting themselves.

This combination of subtle signs from the child with no report of any difficulty from the parent (however concerned a network may be about the family from the known risk factors and general functioning) poses a difficulty for services. How should they delineate levels of need and find ways to respond which will reach the child and the parent-child relationship?

Parents, families and the wider support system

It is appropriate that we support parents who are clearly affected by trauma and adversity in their own right. However, this can bring the optimistic hope that through helping the parent to address their own loss, deprivation and abuse, they will be able to adapt positively to their role as a parent by responding in different ways to their child. Several studies have investigated the progress of a parent's actual emotional and behavioural responses to their child following intervention for their own depression and other difficulties. Parenting interventions have been found to reduce the adult's emotional distress but have not always positively affected outcomes at the level of the child or parent-child relationship (Cox, Puckering, Pound & Mills, 1987).

Murray and colleagues (2003) found that specific interventions including counselling, CBT and psychoanalytical therapies had no significant impact on maternal management of early infant behaviour problems, security of infant/mother attachment, infant cognitive development or any other child outcomes which remained constant at 5 years. Similar findings were reported in a later study by Forman et al. (2007) who included a control group. Half of the parents screened for depression received interpersonal psychotherapy, which had no significant impact on the parent-child relationship or individual child outcomes at follow up.

A robust assessment of the child and parent-child relationship needs to be carried out to shed light on the child's needs in order to inform decision-making and care planning for intervention in a timely way. The timeframe for change to occur in the child's best interest may be lost if a clear profile of the child is not available.

We know the period between birth and 4 years is one of rapid developmental change and consequently services need to be equipped to respond to the varying stages and transitions. Services are therefore often oriented to a specific age group or stage that has an identity of its own, e.g. infancy, toddlerhood, and may be ring-fenced, e.g. a parenting group with entry criteria related to the child's age or specific behaviours, such as toddler tantrums. Age cut-offs are made in an attempt to organise resources effectively but if they are rigid it may be difficult to engage families who present sporadically, resulting in a lack of continuity as services lose knowledge of the family.

A strong, positive case has been made to offer a preventative approach to families by helping vulnerable parents before the baby is born (NICE, 2014). Nevertheless, there remains a need to respond to children in the early years at whatever point the family or child presents, bearing in mind the issues highlighted above.

This is what informed the rationale for the approach developed in the SUSI model spanning the age range of 0–4 years, so that an accurate assessment of the child and parent-child relationship could be delivered as early as possible but one which could also encompass children who are seen later.

It is challenging to provide services for 'hard to reach' families: clear operational inter-agency strategies are required and need to be workable in everyday practice. Issues specific to services for these families relate to ones of definition, but also challenge how we engage and sustain their involvement. There is a continuum, with families who on paper are seen to be in greater need, not always presenting with this at assessment. Parents' lack of insight is prevalent in families with safeguarding concerns. This can affect their view of whether a service may be relevant to them. Barlow, Kirkpatrick, Stewart-Brown & Davies (2005) found that when teenage mothers were interviewed (who had been referred to a support service but had not attended any sessions) they expressed no understanding of the reason for referral.

In the SUSI study one cohort of parents, those engaged with a Parental Mental Health (PMH) service, engaged in part due to their anxiety about the impact of their own mental health on their children. Despite worries whether these could be sensitively addressed, they showed a greater capacity to express concerns. They had already had an experience of being listened to and supported by the PMH team. For families with statutory involvement, a collaborative approach between health, primary and social care can encourage parents to take up the offer of help and create time and space for a specific focus on their relationship with their child. In all clinical services, practitioners need to build trust in the caregivers by a supportive and respectful approach, encouraging them to share their hopes and concerns for their children and their relationships.

The assessment and intervention model developed within community services and trialled in the SUSI study was created to offer a tailored approach to vulnerable families with a wide range of presentations, at different ages and stages. While this is oriented to high risk groups, there are some families where only a brief intervention may be needed. There is an awareness that the work needs to be delivered with flexibility 'on the ground' within the community and networks of which the families are a part. This handbook has been written to describe the work by including the everyday experience of delivering a clinical service to the families in a real, and at times complex, inter-agency community setting.

Notes for this book

- The term 'parent' is used throughout the book to refer to the primary caregiver and attachment figure for the child, whether they are fathers, mothers, wider family members, adoptive or foster parents. Where specific examples describe a particular dyad, this is clarified.
- The case studies used throughout this book are composite examples based on casework; they have been significantly modified to preserve anonymity.
- Permission has been given by parents and professionals for all quotes used in this book.
- Reference is made to resources that were developed during the SUSI project. These include:
  - **handouts** – which provide information for parents on a variety of aspects of social-emotional development in babies and young children, attachment and parenting
  - **homework sheets** – which can be given to parents following interactive sessions for follow-up work (and which they can bring back to next sessions for discussion)
  - **activity templates** – these sheets are composite examples and should be customised to reflect each parent's/child's relationship and situation, and have suggestions which are specific to the child's social-emotional needs.

  All of these resources can be accessed by visiting www.susiweb.co.uk where they can be downloaded and customised to suit personal needs.
- The SUSI model has been cited in the following reviews/reports:
  - 'Achieving emotional well-being for looked after children' (Bazalgette, Rahilly & Trevelyan, 2015) NSPCC
  - 'Looking after infant mental health, our case for change' (2016) NSPCC
  - 'Mapping mental health services for looked after children in London aged 0–5 years' (Moriarty, Baginsky, Gorin, Baginsky & Manthorpe, 2016)
  - Improving mental health support for our children and young people' (2017) Expert Working Group, Social Care Institute for Excellence
  - 'First 1000 days of life inquiry' (2018) Health and Social Care Committee, UK Parliamentary website.

1 Theoretical and research background to the SUSI model

While a large variety of theoretical frameworks contribute to this work, those that have been most relevant to the SUSI model are outlined below.

Infant–child development and infant–parent relationship research

The breadth of research, together with academic and clinical knowledge regarding babies and young children's development and development of the central parent–child relationship is vast. Therefore, we will make reference here to the main fields of which clinicians need to have a working knowledge. A broad base of information on the general developmental stages and the progression of babies and young children's development, including prenatal development, across all domains can be found in numerous works including prenatal development (Brazelton, 1992; Field, 2007; Murray, 2005, 2014; Piontelli, 1992; Stern, 1985).

The caregiving environment

There is rapidly developing evidence about the influence of the caregiving environment on the development of the infant's brain, described and summarised by several notable researchers (McCrory, Gerin & Viding, 2017; Teicher & Samson, 2016).

An extensive and fascinating body of work is captured in several compellingly written and visual narratives (Brazelton, 1974; Murray, 2005; Music, 2017; Stern, 2002; Tronick, 1989). The work explores and highlights:

- the development of the reciprocal relationship between a parent and child, revealing the active contributions from each
- the patterns that emerge including interactive failures and repairs
- the developmental changes over time.

'Intersubjectivity' describes the concept that there is a shared, reciprocal experience between the parent and child whereby the experience of each is having an impact on the experience of the other. Trevarthen and Aitken (2001) observed the way in which even the youngest infants are active in developing co-operative shared activity with their primary caregivers and how successful interactions are supported by the attuned responsiveness of the parent to the baby's initiatives. This is widely viewed as being the basis for all affective interaction, learning and communication. It is being used in applied clinical approaches within attachment and psychoanalytic interventions (Beebe & Lachmann, 2002; Diamond & Marrone, 2003).

In relation to developing problems and more serious psychopathology within parents and babies' relationships, many research studies have provided insights and a means for classifying observable interactions that indicate concern. One of these is the 'AMBIANCE' system (Bronfman, Parsons & Lyons-Ruth, 1999; Haltigan et al., 2019) that looks at atypical maternal behaviours including:

- parental withdrawing response
- negative–intrusive responses
- role confusion responses
- disorientated responses
- affective communication errors.

Longitudinal studies have demonstrated the contribution of these to later psychopathology, with these factors being a greater predictor than measures of infant attachment behaviour alone (Lyons-Ruth, 2008).

Toxic stress

The trauma arising from exposure to chronic adversity has a profound effect on the child at a neurobiological level. It affects their capacity to integrate emotional, cognitive and sensory stimuli in everyday life, as well as manage subsequent stresses that arise. The concept of 'toxic stress' describes a state of intolerable distress in which the child is incapable of regulating their own internal states in the absence of support or containment from a primary carer (the caregiver may also be the source of fear and distress). In these circumstances the child may dissociate (the sensory, cognitive and emotional sensations become fragmented), leaving them unable to comprehend what is happening to them and how they can respond. Where there is insufficient respite from such stress/distress, the child experiences high levels of chronic anxiety, anger and feelings of helplessness. In an effort to ward off further upset or perceived threats, they can react in a similar way to ordinary situations that evoke reminders of past trauma, including neglect. The child may then respond with over-controlling or withdrawn behaviour that may be seen and misunderstood as being 'oppositional' or 'unmotivated'.

Understanding trauma

Experts in the field of complex trauma suggest that childhood trauma, including abuse and neglect, is likely to be one of the greatest public health challenges. They highlight the potential for this to be significantly reduced through effective prevention and intervention (Van der Kolk et al., 2009). The majority of trauma occurs in the family home, therefore the child's own parents or primary caregivers who may be responsible, have themselves frequently been victims of inadequate care or abuse in their early years (Lomanowska, Boivin, Hertzman & Fleming, 2015; Van der Kolk, 2005).

Although these children have experienced multiple traumas and tend to present with complex and varying presentations of developmental delays, the diagnosis of post traumatic stress disorder (PTSD) is no longer considered adequate to describe the exposure to and impact of trauma on the developing child. Children therefore are given a range of co-morbid diagnoses, which often do not reflect the trauma-based experiences or mechanisms that have led to their specific range of problems. The term 'complex trauma' is now used to describe the experience of multiple, repeated and/or chronic 'developmentally adverse traumatic events' which occur in the first few years of life within an interpersonal context (Cook et al., 2005; Van der Kolk, 2005).

A taskforce from the National Child Traumatic Stress Network (NCTSN) has been working to address the need for an adequate diagnosis and has conceptualised the condition 'Developmental Trauma Disorder' (DTD) (Ford et al., 2013)[1]. In her work on trauma, Caroline Garland writes about the 'ways in which traumatic early relationships affect the development of adult personality and vulnerabilities'. When the baby is not protected by sensitive, attuned mothering from 'extreme experiences both environmentally and emotionally' this results in traumatic wounds that shape the child's development and the lasting effects are seen into adulthood (Garland, 1998).

There have been important clinical descriptions of how infants respond to chronic stress, abuse or neglect. In her paper 'Pathological defences in infancy', Fraiberg (1982) describes how these may present in infants. Since then, Lieberman and van Horn (2008) have provided a comprehensive framework for assessing both the child and their relationships. The Diagnostic Classification of Mental Health and Developmental Disorders of Infancy and Early Childhood: Zero to Five (DC: 0–5tm) also gives diagnostic classifications at the individual child level as well as a system for identifying specific relationship presentations (Zero to Three, 2016).

Attachment theory

Attachment refers to the infant's or young child's emotional connection to an adult caregiver – an attachment figure – as inferred from the child's tendency to turn selectively to that adult to increase proximity when needing comfort, support, nurturance or protection.

ZEANAH, BERLIN & BORIS, 2011

Attachment theory, developed by John Bowlby (1969; 1973; 1980), is well known and its theoretical framework is widely used in health, social care and developmental research. It has relevance to work with parents and young children as it demonstrates the effects of early relationship experiences on the child's internal representation of the self and others, developed within specific unique bonds between babies and primary carers.

Attachment, as opposed to other forms of bonds and relationships, is specific to the emotional tie developed between the child and the adult. It is characterised by a tendency to seek and maintain closeness to a special person, especially during times of stress. Another key element to attachment relationships is that it is an enduring tie with one or more specific people. These people are perceived to offer safety, comfort and pleasure; therefore the loss or perceived loss of the person will cause anxiety and distress (Zeanah, Berlin & Boris, 2011).

Along with the biologically and emotionally driven need to seek contact and gain comfort from specific caregivers, there is a parallel exploratory system at work. This system enables the child to begin to separate and move away from the adult in order to explore the environment. These two systems of attachment and exploration are balanced in the presence of an emotionally available caregiver creating the 'secure base' experience (Bowlby, 1988).

Attachment and future relationships

Attachment research has combined an understanding of how early relationships shape the mind (internal world) and behaviour of the developing child in many areas of their functioning. These include emotional regulation, social relatedness and the capacity to gradually integrate their personal experiences into a coherent narrative (Sroufe, 2005). Understanding the contribution that attachment relationships bring to both outward behavioural responses, as well as the child's autobiographical memory and sense of self, helps us to reflect on the impact of the primary caregiving bond on a child's external as well as internal world. Not only do securely attached children have trust in attachment figures and later in people more widely, they also learn to trust their own understanding and views of the world and situations they face day to day. Unsurprisingly, with this greater self-awareness and the belief that others can help them when needed, they also have a more advanced capacity to communicate than insecurely attached children, regarding both their physiological and emotional states (Cichetti & White, 1990). Conversely, in clinical contexts it is common to observe how frequently some babies and young children do not express their wishes or needs directly.

Patterns of secure/insecure attachment

There are three 'organised' patterns of secure and insecure attachment:

- secure
- insecure-avoidant
- insecure-ambivalent.

These 'organised' patterns were formulated by Ainsworth (1978) and added to later by Mary Main, who introduced the category of disorganised attachment (Main & Solomon, 1986). These classifications are important in terms of the common patterns of child and adult behavioural and emotional responses within each category. Amongst others, Cassidy (1994) describes how the child adapts to the parent's state of mind in relation to their own experience of attachment, emotional regulation and trauma. For example, the 'avoidant' parent often denies any negative characteristics of their own childhood, yet they may withdraw if the baby expresses negative emotion, and will not respond to the infant's bids for comfort. This in turn can cause the baby to develop an avoidance strategy, with predominantly neutral affect and an absence of signalling distress when separated. This helps to minimise the emotional demands on the parent and maintain the 'status quo' of the parent's state of mind: in effect the baby learns to help the parent out, rather than being able to rely on an adult to help regulate their own emotional states.

Despite there being risks to the child who has adopted these strategies, the insecure classification of 'anxious avoidant' or 'anxious ambivalent' is not predictive or synonymous with a clinical disorder as such. However, there can be longer term consequences affecting an individual's capacity to develop positive relationships with peers and adults, to be adaptable and resilient, and to have self-control and tolerate uncertainty (Ramsdal, Bergvik & Wynn, 2015)[2].

In the clinical context, a high proportion of children referred to CAMHS present with disorganised attachments (Green, Stanley & Peters, 2007). Awareness of how a developing disorganised attachment may manifest itself is important and needs rigorous observations and careful formulation if the classification term is to be used. It may be more appropriate and helpful clinically to describe the signs of disorganised responses, including dissociation, which may only present in fleeting moments, such as a disturbed or distorted facial expression or contradictory odd movements.

Lieberman & Pawl (1990) formulated three clinical disorders of attachment that could be identified once the child has turned one year old. These are distinguishable by the distorted imbalance between the attachment and exploratory systems. These clinical descriptions are especially helpful as they fit with the contradictory patterns of difficulties or symptoms in the children who are commonly seen in the clinic or in outreach home visits.

Psychoanalytic theory

Sigmund Freud

Freud developed psychoanalytic theory as a way of understanding the meaning and complexity of human needs, impulses, motivation and desire. He acknowledged the importance of the child's experience in early infancy and how this shapes their future development. Freud noticed the interplay between biology and psychology in the infant's relationship to, and identification with, their mother. He famously wrote 'the ego is first and foremost a bodily ego: it is not merely a surface entity but is itself the projection of a surface' (1923), meaning that the baby's feelings and experiences are first and foremost felt in their body.

During the second half of the twentieth century, the work of three more remarkable psychoanalysts profoundly affected the way we think about children and their relationship needs. Much of our current thinking and practice has been influenced by their work, leading to changes in childcare.

John Bowlby

John Bowlby was the founder of Attachment theory. His work brought about influential changes in the way children are treated when they are hospitalised. Previously, a familiar caregiver was not permitted to stay with the child, which caused great distress. Bowlby and colleagues studied these reactions to 'abandonment' and lobbied for a change that would allow the caregiver to remain with the child, as he felt this sort of experience was one that could give rise to an 'insecure' attachment. While particularly pertinent in situations of hospitalisation, this was also applicable to any separation that was experienced as abandonment.

Donald Winnicott

Donald Winnicott was a paediatrician who noticed that many of his child patients' troubled behaviour was closely linked to distress in the parent. Winnicott famously said, 'There is no such thing as a baby' as well as 'a baby alone doesn't exist'. He went on to assert that what does exist is always a 'nursing couple', i.e. a baby plus someone who takes care of him/her (1960). Therefore, the mother's (or carer's) state of mind has a large part to play in how the baby first experiences the world around him/her.

Anna Freud

Anna Freud came to London with her father, Sigmund Freud, in 1938. After his death, she set up the Hampstead War Nurseries in 1941 to care for children traumatised by the war, loss and separations. She was able to study the ways in which it had affected them. Her later work was shaped by this experience. She collaborated with another psychoanalyst and a lawyer to publish *Beyond the Best Interests of the Child* (1973) which heralded the idea that a child has legal rights as an individual.

Other psychoanalysts who have made significant contributions to our understanding of individual psychological development are outlined below.

Erik Erickson

Erickson (1965) expanded Freud's emphasis on individual development in his eight stages of psychosocial development. He more clearly linked the move from the infant's total need and dependency upon the primary carer to their developmental move to phases of separateness and individuation.

As the child moves through developmental phases, what happens internally is partly influenced by the responses they receive from the world around them. Failures in responses from parents, environment or society can lead to disturbances in later life. In *The Psychological Birth of the Human Infant* by Mahler, Pine and Bergman (1975), their description of work with infants and toddlers from 6 months to 3 years captures the importance of the child's experience of their body as central to their development of separateness from their primary carer/love object.

Melanie Klein and Hanna Segal

The work of Klein[3] (1928) and Segal (1964) further enriches our understanding of the infant's anxieties and fantasies as they develop an awareness of separateness: 'me/not me'. Increased understanding of the early psychic development and mechanisms, including the centrality of the infant's body in 'holding and experiencing' their feelings, are crucial in understanding the exciting and challenging terrain that the infant faces and the need for love and support to negotiate these challenges.

Throughout our clinical work, some babies, infants and toddlers were seen who 'stiffened' their bodies, or turned their faces away in response to being held, or in response to a certain look or tone of voice from the parent or primary carer. The tense, emotionally painful experiences became lodged, not only in their minds but in their bodies and were experienced by the baby or toddler as a whole body/feeling experience, contributing to their internal and external blueprint.

Wilfred Bion

Bion (1962b) developed his ideas by building on those of Melanie Klein about projection and projective identification. In relation to the work described in this book, of particular interest is his concept of ‘containment’. It is an idea involving two individuals: the ‘container’ and the ‘contained’. In those situations, where the parent (referred to as ‘mother’ for the remainder of this section) has had little or no containment from their own caregiver, they will find it hard to provide this for their baby and it is the therapist who initially becomes the ‘container’ and provides it for both. The therapist’s role (container) is to observe the behaviour of mother and baby/child, to be in touch emotionally with what is passing between them, and to put into words what is happening. By demonstrating that she can *feel and think* about the situation, the therapist shows the mother how to be in touch with her baby’s experiences and will explore the mother’s own emotional responses to her baby’s behaviour or demeanour. With time and repeated experiences, the mother (contained) will become identified with the therapist’s capacity to contain and be able to take on board her own and her baby’s distress or delight: in that way, the mother can share the experience with the baby as the therapist is sharing it with her.

This is particularly important in relation to frightening fantasies, such as abandonment, or angry, hateful feelings of frustration. This reflective process diminishes the fearful aspects of the relationship: the baby grasps that the mother is not frightened, and the mother calms the baby. Through projective identification, the mother’s experience of the therapist’s function becomes her own, so eventually she is able to provide the containing function for herself and for her baby. Through the early months of life this pattern is repeated many times over, and as the baby develops s/he learns to provide some of this for themself (just as the mother has done) and is able to calm themself.

Two particularly helpful psychoanalytic concepts relevant to this work are described below.

Transference

A core psychoanalytic framework within which several concepts can be understood revolve around the theory of an individual having an internal world as well as an experience of the external world. It is understood that mental processes occur between these two. Psychoanalytic thinking and theoretical constructs can help us to understand some of the underlying, unconscious dynamics affecting both the relationship between parent and child, as well as their responses to ourselves as professionals: the latter being referred to as the 'transference'. This is a process of actualisation of unconscious wishes or fears in the present, although it is related to significant people or situations in the past.

Parents, and to some extent children who may be toddler-aged and above, bring their internal representations and expectations of 'parental' figures to the relationship with the therapist. The 'transference' may be enacted in both positive and negative ways.

Parents who have experienced abuse, unpredictability and lack of care themselves are often suspicious and fearful of professionals which 'makes the ordinary client-professional relationship a first step to be achieved rather than to be taken for granted' (Bentovim, 1980).

Positive transference from the parent to the therapist, as someone who is trying to make things better for their baby, often runs in parallel with a negative transference. Within the negative transference, the therapist may be experienced as untrustworthy, unhelpful or unavailable. This happens when memories and feelings are triggered during the parent-infant/child work associated with emotional vulnerability, rage or fear from their own early childhood. Understanding these identifications, which may occur from the parent towards the child, and separately with the therapist, are important and need to be reflected on outside the clinical sessions in supervision or case reviews. Clinical decisions can then be made about whether it is appropriate to address the transference more directly or not. These decisions are based on the clinical experience and background of the therapist and the mental and emotional state of the parent.

In most psychotherapeutic approaches to parent-child therapy, there is also a strong focus on developmental guidance. Through this, there is the obvious benefit for the child of having a more attuned, informed parent, as well as the positive aspect of the therapeutic relationship that can develop through this support.

Countertransference

Countertransference describes the emotional states evoked in the therapist from the adult or child's projections, the cause of which may not be immediately obvious. This can be used as a clinical tool in psychotherapeutic work to understand more of the underlying communications from the individual that are not being directly expressed. Feelings experienced by the therapist as a negative countertransference could include irritation, being paralysed, unable to think, and within supervision this can be considered in order to understand what aspects of the individual are being brought to the therapeutic process.

Specific to the field of infant mental health, Selma Fraiberg, Professor of Child Psychoanalysis, described the notion of the 'ghosts' that may be found in families 'which compel the repetition of the past in the present'. In her clinical work, Fraiberg showed that some parents, despite wishing their children to have a better childhood experience than their own, were not able to put this into practice because unconscious representations of the past were impacting on their feelings and behaviour toward their child. She wrote: 'while none has issued an invitation, the ghosts take up residence and conduct the rehearsal of the family tragedy from a tattered script' (Fraiberg, Adelson & Shapiro, 1975).

As not all parents who had a neglectful or abusive past re-enact the same with their own child, Fraiberg examined the ways in which parents responded to their own previous experiences of adversity. Two defences used by parents were linked to an inability to protect and separate their children from their own painful past: parents who showed denial of affect associated with previous trauma; and parents who identified with the perpetrator of their own abuse.

Many other therapists and academics (Cowan, Callaghan, Kan & Richardson, 2015; Fonagy, Steele, Moran, Steele & Higgitt, 1993; Hopkins, 1992) have presented research and clinical evidence of the need to consider the intergenerational transmission of trauma that can adversely impact on the infant–parent relationship, when the baby represents an attribute of the parent's self that is disowned or rejected, or when the baby comes to represent a significant figure in the parent's own past.

Systems and ecological theory

Systemic ideas have contributed to a framework which holds the view that problems may be seen as interpersonal rather than individual. This means that an individual's experience and identity is shaped through the interaction, communication and relationships with others (Dallos & Draper, 2010).

Systemic psychotherapy and family therapy, like most forms of family counselling, are based on systems theory. Family therapy contends that the internal dynamics of the family system can produce and sustain problematic behaviours in a family member. On a wider level, systems theory has helped practitioners and agencies consider the influence of relationships from within the extended family, community and professional networks, and supports the notion of utilising the strengths and resources therein.

Stressors

Based on attachment theory and neuroscientific findings, it is known that many individual risk factors might predispose a child to poor psychological well-being, or to being more vulnerable to mental health problems. However, the cumulative environmental impact of the system surrounding the child needs to be considered. Bronfenbrenner's ecological systems model speaks to the fact that children's difficulties do not occur in a vacuum. The children and parents in the more 'vulnerable' populations have a higher than average number of social and environmental stressors impacting upon them (Bronfenbrenner, 1979; Coman & Devaney, 2011).

Large scale epidemiological studies on urban stress and mental health have found that stressors on children's mental health include families' socio-economic status, childhood poverty, parental separations, adult relationships dominated by violence and arguments, and physical ill-health (Langner & Michael, 1963). Economically disadvantaged children are exposed to more environmental stressors which have a negative impact on their well-being which decreases future opportunities (Evans, 2004). Evans utilises a systemic approach and puts forward the view that the 'pathological' part of childhood poverty may be due to the cumulative effect of environmental risk factors.

Adversity and deprivation – defensive responses in systems

The impact of adversity and deprivation for individuals is known to be felt within the wider system around children and their families. The NICE guidance for LAC (2010), together with the 'Every Child Matters' (Department for Education and Skills, ECM, 2003) policy document, recommend having a strong network in place to co-ordinate the support for the individual child and their primary caregivers.

Theorists have offered the view that both the child and/or the parent's past experiences of maltreatment and neglect are so powerful that these unprocessed feelings are felt within the system at large, creating defensive responses in parts of the multi-agency network. The responses often reflect re-enactments of the primitive dynamics within the birth family, and can paralyse those working within the system (Britton, 1981; Heimann, 1950). One example of this might be an inability to think about the child's needs and could be considered to reproduce an act of neglect towards the child, a concept termed the 'triple-deprivation' of children in care (Emanuel, 2006). However, research in the field has demonstrated that, particularly in crisis situations, staff may have limited capacity to engage with collaborative and systemic work (Darlington, Feeney & Rixon, 2005).

---

1 The trials to date have found support for the hypothesised symptom structure of developmental trauma disorder (DTD) which describes distinct but related domains of dysregulation that include: emotion/physiological; cognitive/behavioural; and interpersonal/self-identity in the context of attachment and interpersonal trauma. This diagnosis is yet to be included in the psychiatric classifications (DSM-V and ICD-11) although a strong case was made for this diagnosis to be established. The National Child Traumatic Stress Network (NCTSN) ran a field trial and found that 'a diagnosis of DTD was significantly predicted by traumatic attachment disruptions in childhood, especially when those disruptions were accompanied by experiences of interpersonal victimization' (Trauma Center at Justice Resource Institute, 2012). Complex post traumatic stress disorder (CPTSD) has been included as a diagnostic category in the International Classification of Diseases, 11th Edition, consisting of six symptom clusters: the three PTSD criteria of re-experiencing, avoidance and hyper-vigilance, in addition to three disturbances of self-organisation (DSO) symptoms defined as emotional dysregulation, interpersonal difficulties and negative self-concept (Jowett, Karatzias, Shevlin & Albert, 2020). In the babies and very young children seen in the pilot and SUSI studies, as well as within our LAC clinical mental health service, we have identified a high prevalence of

symptoms associated with DTD, albeit some in the early stages of formation. Signs of developmental trauma can manifest in subtle and/or fleeting presentations at times in such young children and may be even more prone to being missed or misunderstood than in school-age children and adolescents. This phenomenon was highlighted in an independent research report by The Childhood Wellbeing Research Centre. This gave a comprehensive review of the research and literature on neglect, in order to raise awareness and inform practice for professionals making assessments regarding the severity of neglect, perhaps the most confusing form of child maltreatment, in order to consider the current and future impact on the child. The report draws attention to the need to observe what may be missing from parent–child interactions and relationships, seen in the behaviours of both child and parent, e.g. a quiet passive baby, a parent that does not notice or respond to the baby. It also helps us to think about how practitioners may be drawn more towards the needs of a vulnerable adult parent, which may then influence their perspective on the child's needs and whether sufficient change is being made (Brandon et al., 2014).

2 Insecure and disorganised attachments have been shown in numerous studies to be associated with a range of poorer outcomes, including later psychopathology (Green & Goldwyn, 2002; Van IJzendoorn, Schuengel & Bakermans-Kranenburg, 1999), externalising disorders (i.e. conduct and behaviour problems), (Fearon, Bakermans-Kranenburg, Van IJzendoorn, Lapsley, & Roisman, 2010) and personality disorder (Steele & Siever, 2010). Along with the greater vulnerability that an insecure attachment may bring to a context of psychosocial adversity, conversely secure attachments can help to protect the child's brain and developmental progress in the face of exposure to traumatic stress (Glaser, 2014).

3 Kleinian theory is built on ideas about how the infant experiences their first relationship with a caregiver. This relationship is modified over time from a primitive split between 'good' and 'bad' objects, to more complex acceptance of objects as an amalgam of both.

For this to happen, the caregiver needs to be attuned to the infant's experiences of frustrations and fears, so that the infant is helped to tolerate the 'bad' and return to less hateful states of mind. Similarly, the caregiver needs to give the infant enough experiences that promote 'loving' states of mind, so that the possibility of 'good' experiences can be trusted. Klein called the primitive split state the 'paranoid/schizoid' state of mind, and she called the more complex integrated state the 'depressive' position. They are not static. These internal states of mind are usually unconscious, but nevertheless in adulthood they have a profound effect on our relationships. When a state of mind cannot be tolerated by an individual, that person tries to rid themselves of it by 'projecting' it, thereby seeing the world around, or others, as 'hateful', rather than experiencing the hate themselves.

2 The model in practice

The SUSI work was a great resource – it made a real difference to the families for someone to offer targeted and focused interventions without judgement.

PARENTAL MENTAL HEALTH WORKER

This chapter describes the design and structure of the SUSI model. It outlines briefly each stage of the process and how it can be delivered practically in a clinical setting. The clinical work is described in greater detail in Chapters 4, 5 and 6. The research study itself is described in more detail in Chapter 10 but aspects of it will be referred to here as there was much to be learned from delivering a clinical approach within a research protocol. This has subsequently influenced the clinical service that is offered.

Origins of the SUSI project

This parent-child therapeutic work has evolved over the past 25 years in an inner London borough. The clinical teams have had a remit to offer assessment and therapeutic services to babies and young children under the age of five, along with their parents and primary caregivers. These services include a community under 5s team serving the local generic population, together with a targeted looked after and adopted children's mental health service (CAMHS) where the clinical research took place over the past 10 years. The model has been trialled in two separate studies (Hardy & Murphy, 2013; Hardy et al., 2015; Hardy & Murphy, 2018). Populations using the clinical services experience many kinds of adversity including poor parental mental health, domestic violence, poverty, and drug and alcohol misuse, with the children having experienced or being vulnerable to abuse, neglect and trauma.

Experts in the Infant Mental Health and Early Years fields (Fraiberg, 1994; Lieberman & Van Horn, 2008; Stern, 1985; Zeanah, Berlin & Boris, 2011) provided practitioners and clinical researchers with rich evidence and conceptual frameworks which informed and inspired direct work with families in recent decades. Our understanding of the particular ways in which young children's social-emotional vulnerability may present has been greatly helped by this. Nonetheless, the translation of these ideas into everyday practice remains a challenge.

Our clinical experience of offering a service to one of the most high-risk groups of children in society, i.e. looked after children (LAC), made us aware that many of the children referred to our service had been displaying signs of difficulty at an earlier age. Indicators of these problems arose when taking a detailed history as part of their assessment. This in turn stimulated our ideas to develop a pilot project (Hardy et al., 2015) that would involve assessing the youngest babies and children (0–4 year olds) as soon as they first became looked after. Ideas regarding this were supported by the new joint National Institute for Health and Care Excellence (NICE) and Social Care Institute for Excellence (SCIE) (2010) guidance for LAC that was being finalised at the time. The recommendations stated that there should be an assessment of needs for all babies and young children who become looked after. This would ensure access to specialist services and further highlighted the need to ensure that carers and frontline practitioners working with babies and young children would receive specialist training.

Having successfully introduced the assessment approach in the pilot study with under 5s looked after children in 2010–11, we extended the target groups in our second study (SUSI) to three high risk cohorts in the community to include:

1. children of parents referred to the Parental Mental Health (PMH) team
2. children new to a Child Protection Plan
3. newly looked after children (as in the pilot study)

The following indicators from the pilot study demonstrated that a longer intervention was required in many cases:

- the significant levels of social-emotional and attachment needs identified
- the clinical presentations of the child over time.

Thus the rationale for the SUSI study was established.

An accessible model

The approach taken in the SUSI study of targeting children and families that have known risk factors for the child and parent–child relationship is one possible model for a clinical service in a community multi-agency setting. It reaches out to children who are not typically being referred to CAMHS or other Early Help services and can avoid the need for referrals. It addresses the difficulties for professionals identifying and then articulating these difficulties in a way that would facilitate entry to a CAMHS or specialist under 5s service.

The assessment and intervention were designed to be integrated within a multi-agency service model with clear operational links in place. Concerns regarding children can be escalated in consultation with the network where joint planning regarding intervention and/or care plans is made together with referral to other services as appropriate.

The design of the clinical model was created to address the challenges of:

- identifying and articulating concerns about babies and young children's social–emotional development
- engaging parents and caregivers of children from vulnerable populations
- acceptance of the clinical approach within the wider family and multi-agency network.

Key features and solutions included:

1. flexible delivery of location and timing
2. tailored intervention for child and family
3. transparent links and time-points for inter-agency feedback and liaison.

1 Accessibility and flexible delivery

Offering flexibility around the location and timing of meetings was important from the initial engagement of families through to the intervention and review stages. The therapists, key workers and the family considered which locations would be acceptable and least stressful. Some parents were happy to meet in their home, while others preferred to meet in a community setting. Times of meetings also required planning and flexibility on the part of the therapists. The many and varied demands and stressors on the

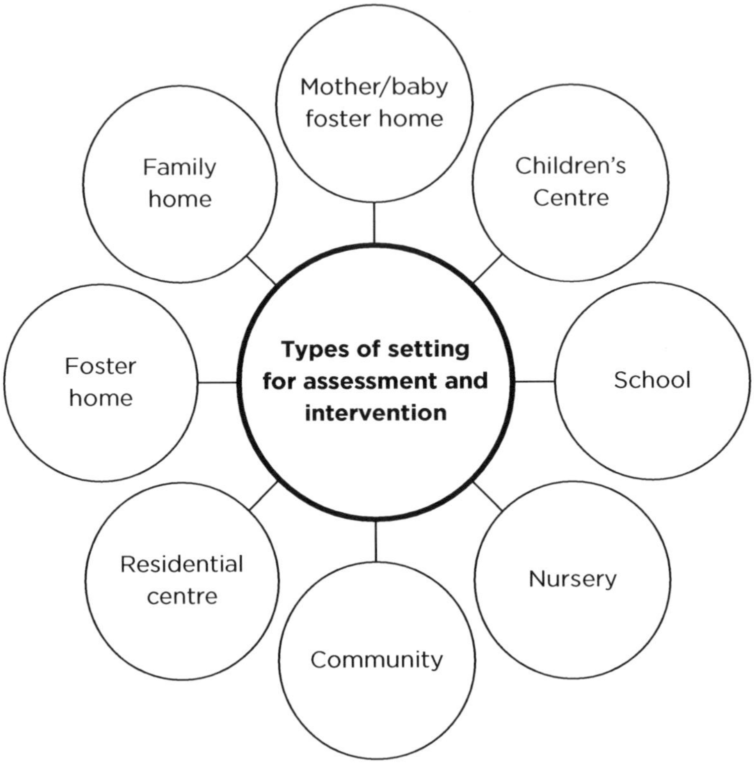

Figure 2.1 Assessment and intervention could take place in a number of settings, according to each family's preference

families were recognised. The burden of time/effort on families undertaking the assessment was also considered. The number of assessment measures was limited, as was the timeframe (to two visits generally).

The model needed to be delivered in a variety of locations and it also had to be adapted to a range of different parent–child dyads. We had experience of working with caregivers who were at different stages of their relationship with their child, for instance, some just getting to know one another and others with more established relationships, e.g. children new to foster carers, with birth parents or kinship relatives, and adoptive parents. At the assessment stage this had many implications. Taking a developmental history had to be approached differently according to the child's contact and history with their parent, e.g. if the parent had post-natal health problems, or the child experienced prenatal adversity, disruptions or separations in the early months.

2 Tailored intervention

Each intervention was adapted to the individual child and their relationship to their primary caregiver(s) and was informed by the assessment. Reasons for an intervention being offered were outlined in straightforward but sensitive language in the assessment report and feedback discussion with parents and caregivers. Core components of the intervention are described in the SUSI process section below. The choice and ideas about the initial focus of the intervention was discussed with the family following the assessment and examples of this are outlined in Chapter 4. At a practical level, it was vital that appointments were made at times and in locations that the family could manage.

Tailoring of the intervention has made this work applicable to a wide variety of caregiver–child relationships, including birth and non-birth parents, as well as long- and short-term caregivers.

3 Inter-agency liaison and communication

Support for parents from their existing network of family, friends and professionals was utilised to help set up joint meetings where the parents had the choice of who they would like to join them. This was important in helping the parent to feel more comfortable and confident, with their support person being able to raise issues and seek clarity about the work we were offering. Where parents had some difficulty in retaining or processing information, mental capacity issues needed to be addressed before meeting them and advice and clarification sought from their own support network, including legal representation where applicable.

Informal feedback with families was appropriate for many parents in the community when they could decide who they would like to be part of feedback and future meetings. Lots of work was put into creating opportunities for contact with fathers, partners and other important family members so they could be involved in the assessment and intervention at all stages of the process.

For families that had existing professional networks or statutory involvement, it was important that direct liaison was inbuilt into the SUSI process with agreed time-points for sharing information and planning meetings. This would take place with the parents at existing forums, e.g. Team Around the Child (TAC), Core Group meetings, LAC reviews. In addition, there was a need for smaller, more sensitive meetings with parents where a detailed discussion of the child or the parent–child relationship could take place; subsequently this information was fed into more formal decision-making forums.

The SUSI process

This section will briefly describe the core components of SUSI, from the initial engagement of families to follow-up reviews. All of the stages were followed within the SUSI study. This may be relevant to some clinical services while others may utilise sections of the model as a stand-alone approach, for instance, the first three stages from engagement through to feedback of the assessment.

Pathways for the identification of children and parents needing assessment should be determined at a local community and inter-agency level, with practical systems in place for families to access a clinical team. Suggestions for how this can be adapted to different contexts are described in subsequent chapters.

Engagement

Ways in which engagement with parents and children was facilitated, with generic ideas and some examples from our clinical service and the SUSI project, are considered below.

Whether the assessment was being offered in a mainstream service or research/project context, there needed to be a reliable source of information about the families with children that met a higher risk threshold. Once identified by colleagues in partner agencies, the process of engaging the parents began. Information from key workers guided this early stage and consideration was given to how and where to meet face to face with parents to start a discussion. Meetings often included a key worker and/or family member.

There was a need to present the model to parents in a clear way, while not overwhelming them with too much information. A variety of written and visual materials were prepared that were relevant to the local context and shared with parents in these initial discussions. Along with discussion, the resources were helpful in illustrating the aims and stages of the input as well as the manner and timetable for sharing information, e.g. GP letters, reports to Children's Social Care when there was statutory involvement. Sometimes

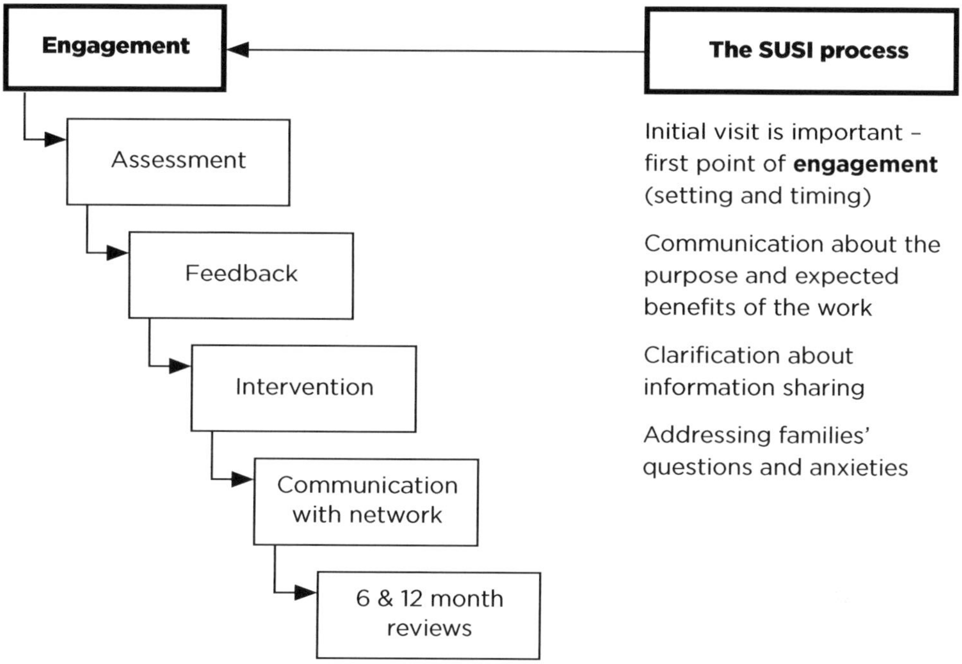

Figure 2.2 The first step was to engage with the families

this required a couple of meetings so the family could reflect on the detail and the implications for them and their child, e.g. sharing of an assessment where a Child Protection Plan was in place.

For many parents it can be daunting to think about a significant commitment to any service, even when delivered flexibly. It seemed helpful for parents to be clear that they could be involved on a step-by-step basis, so they had choice and control over their involvement. For example, it was reassuring that the initial stage of assessment consisted of two visits followed by a feedback session, at which point they could review their position. The availability of an intervention from the same team, should this be indicated from the assessment, contributed to many families viewing the offer as relevant and helpful, and seemed an important factor in their engagement.

Assessment

An assessment approach was chosen that combined standardised measures, history taking and clinical observations to gain a rounded picture of the child's social-emotional and general development in the context of difficulties but also the strengths in the parent-child relationship. The parent's physical and mental health, together with their social and cultural context, contributed to our understanding and formulation of the issues. These were summarised in a short report for families. It was recognised that aspects could be challenging, e.g. the unstructured play observation for many parents and carers, therefore the measures were selected carefully so that parents and children could complete the process.

Flexibility in how the measures and clinical discussion/observation were delivered was important. Many families used the choice they had as to which aspects of the assessment to undertake at each visit, e.g. if the parent-child free play observation was planned but the child was tired/distressed we could reschedule and do informal observations, discussion or other standardised measures instead.

It was recognised that the backdrop of mental health and/or complex trauma, and intergenerational adversity in many of the families, led to concerns that they may be judged or criticised. The assessment inevitably touched on difficult, painful and sensitive issues, and parents needed to express these in their own time and at their own pace. As the narratives of the family's experience and history required time to be told, it was important to remember that the team could be working with a number of unknowns or family secrets. Carrying out work to address and alleviate difficulties in the present should run in parallel to hearing more of a family's history.

Clinical observations of the child and their interaction with the parent, and with therapists, gives us insights and hypotheses about a child's underlying emotional states. In the early stages of getting acquainted it is noted that the child's communications can be subtle if they are quiet and unresponsive, self-reliant and 'keeping busy'. Children often let us know their worries and upsets without words: showing stress in somatic, behavioural, regulatory and social-emotional presentations. As part of the clinical observation, the absence of the child's responses which would be expected in a given situation was noted, e.g. not crying when their parent left the room or when they hurt themselves, or not responding to social cues to look and respond to another person.

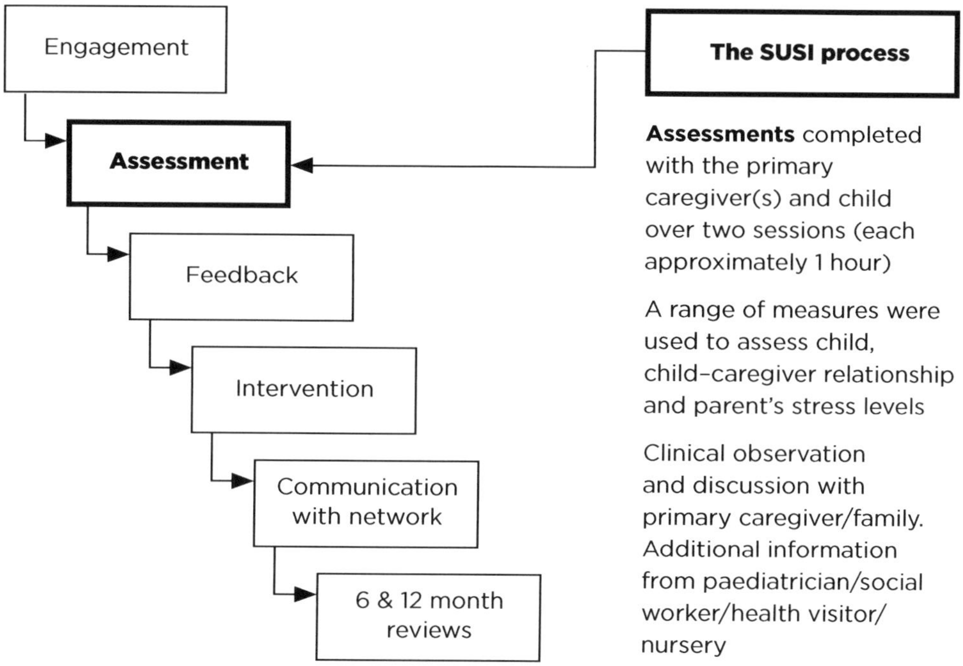

Figure 2.3 Assessment stage

Feedback

The feedback stage of the model (which is described in more detail in Chapter 4) helped to find common ground and a shared language when talking about difficulties and strengths in the child's presentation and the parent–child relationship. The first steps for the tailored intervention were then agreed. The written reports were brief and avoided professional jargon, bringing the child's experience to the fore. They were also written with sensitivity to the challenges faced by parents, acknowledging the efforts they had made. A template for the written report can be found at the end of Chapter 4 (page 93). This can be adapted to different clinical and inter-agency contexts.

Everyday clinical practice shows the need for the assessment content and resulting recommendations to be accessible and meaningful to busy families and professionals. Both groups may be thinking about the child's needs

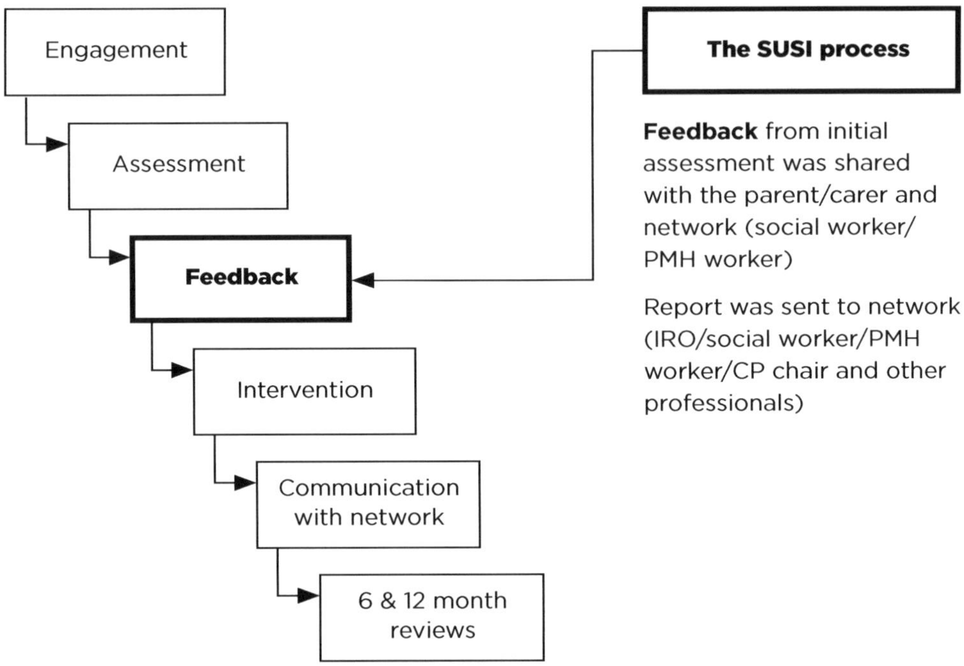

Figure 2.4 Feedback of assessment

in a new light for the first time. Therefore, the child's parent(s) as well as their network needed to be engaged in considering further exploration and action. This needed a sensitive approach with discussion of some initial aims, drawn from the individual formulation within the assessment.

Intervention

Due to the widely varying contexts for the child, and the different stages of relationships with parents/carers (from age to care status), the intervention used a range of techniques/approaches. However, all were specifically targeted to the parent-child relationship as the main agent for change. (These are described in detail in Chapter 5.)

An essential component was an understanding of the parents' experience of the child and their relationship, which began in the assessment and continued to be supported and explored throughout the intervention. Within the SUSI study, a short- to medium-term approach was provided, with 15 sessions for birth parents/kinship or adoptive parents and 10 sessions for

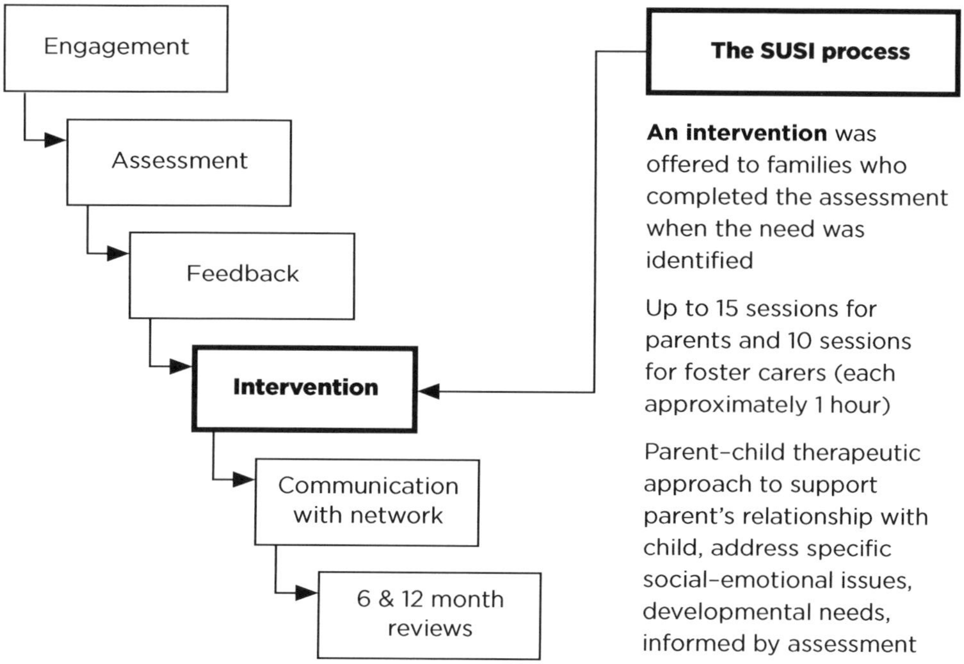

Figure 2.5 Intervention stage

foster carers. The structure and delivery of each intervention was informed by the assessment and included a combination of:

- parent-child relationship 'live' work:
  - using spontaneous interactions in play-based sessions (structured and/or non-directive)
  - a focus on specific communications and interactions that are adaptive and promote the parent-child relationship
  - promoting parental thoughtfulness through exploration of the child's specific responses and behaviours that signal the child's underlying mental and emotional states
  - addressing maladaptive patterns of interaction
- reflective discussion with parents:
  - discussion of current experiences of parenting and relationship with their child
  - exploring links between past and present experiences that relate to the relationship and the child's needs

- liaison and joint work with network:
  - shared understanding of the child's needs with the wider family and/or network
  - discussions to develop a multi-agency care plan as needed.

Intervention themes were created to serve as a guide to important topics to be used alongside the therapeutic techniques. They describe core aspects and dynamics of parent–child relationships, e.g.:

- the attachment system
- parent's attunement to their child's signals
- autonomy
- joint attention
- emotional regulation.

A full description can be found in Chapter 6.

The themes were incorporated in a flexible way to respond to the emotional states of the child and family. Some had more resonance for families than others and could be used accordingly across several sessions. As the intervention progressed, different approaches were introduced if they became relevant and clinically useful to the child and family. For example, the decision about when to bring in the theme of how a parent's 'buttons get pressed' would vary according to how much a parent could reflect on their emotional responses (and past experience) in the parent–child live work.

Communication with the network

At a service and inter-agency level, it was essential that a new clinical model was embedded in the complex network around children and families. It was also important that this service innovation was 'acceptable' to other professionals and agencies. Partner agencies needed to see the model as relevant to their target populations. It was also important that the implementation methods were in tune with existing operational practices and decision-making procedures that were part of agencies' everyday working practice. (See Chapter 3 and Chapter 8 for more detailed descriptions of the integration of the model within a range of community services for adults and children.)

Clear time-points for formal feedback and communication were embedded in the SUSI process. These were discussed at the initial meetings with parents and professionals so the type and timing of information-sharing

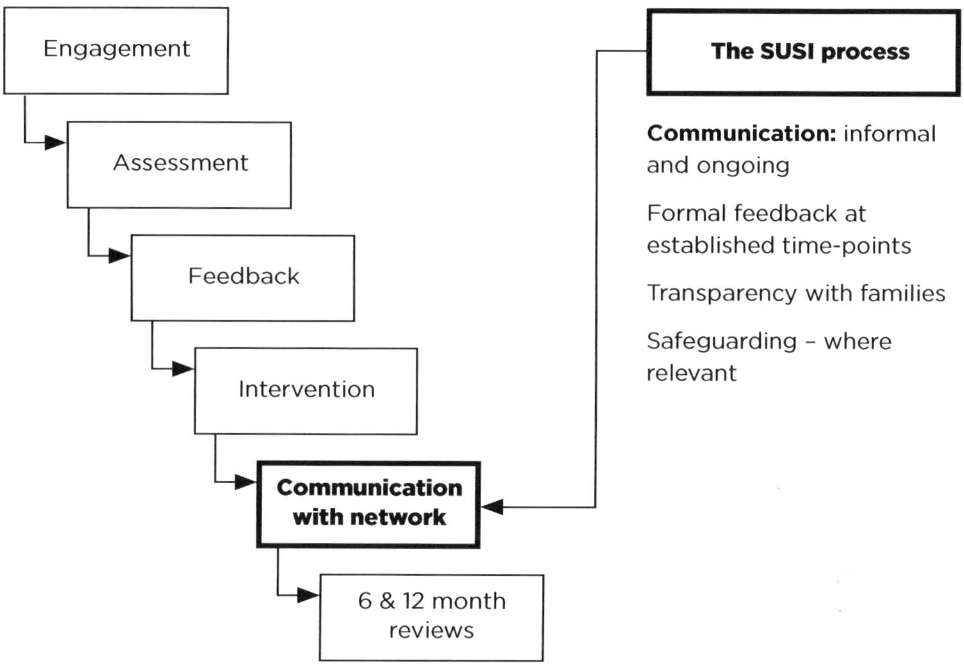

Figure 2.6 Communication with the family's network

was transparent. For example, families were aware that their child's GP would be contacted at regular intervals, and that the assessment and review reports would be shared with Social Care if they had statutory involvement. Depending on the need of the child and family, or changes in the network, additional reviews were also arranged as necessary. Joint meetings were scheduled with families during the work when there were specific concerns or changes to the plan.

Throughout the SUSI work, whether in a project or clinical service, other professionals or family members were included as much as possible. When parents were considering taking part, colleagues in primary care or education (health visitor, nursery worker) or adult services (AMH practitioner or voluntary worker) who had an existing positive relationship would be invited to join initial meetings. This was an opportunity to discuss any concerns the parents might have in relation to the work with a known, trusted person present, and the team could get to know the family's network better.

Figure 2.7 Follow-up reviews

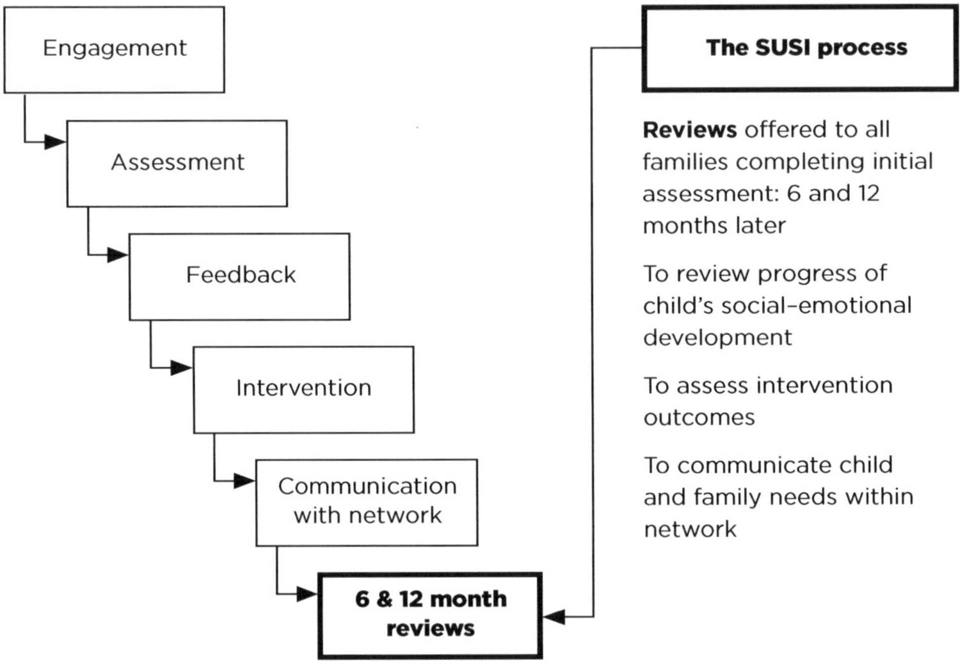

Follow-up reviews

Within the SUSI study, follow-up reviews took place at 6- and 12-month time-points, when the measures and clinical assessment were repeated. While the aims included the assessment of intervention outcomes and the progress review of the child's social-emotional development, there were other benefits that had relevance to a clinical service. Many families were keen to meet again and have the chance to reflect on their child's well-being and changes they had made in their relationship. There was also the opportunity to consider a new developmental phase the child was moving into and to support the parent's confidence in approaching this.

For other families who were facing challenges, other services might be engaged as appropriate, depending on whether the focus for input was required for the adult or child. With parent's agreement, meetings and/or liaison with the family's network took place to provide recommendations or practical advice from the review assessment's findings.

3 Getting started

The SUSI project meant that our young babies had an early intervention from a therapist that they would not have received otherwise, as they wouldn't have met thresholds.

SOCIAL WORKER

It is important when developing any new services to consider previous and existing reports/reviews in the borough (inspections, public health reviews, etc.) to learn what the main issues are and to consider how best to work with partner agencies to address the problems. These include:

- Children's Social Care (CSC)
- Child Health
- Adult Mental Health (AMH)
- Children's Centres
- Universal services including health visiting
- Child and Adolescent Mental Health (CAMHS)
- Education and colleagues in the voluntary sector.

This chapter starts by describing the relationships and links that were built with partner agencies. It outlines the systems that were created for clinical governance, information sharing, training and recruitment of staff. Practical examples from the SUSI project are also described, which may be useful for those wishing to develop similar services.

Engaging and informing local stakeholders

It is evident that many agencies are involved when working with families. While multiple sources of information may be useful, it can also delay decision-making that is sensitive to the needs of the child. Some of the complexities around these issues will be dealt with further in Chapter 8. In this chapter, we will focus on the need to become familiar with other agencies' working models, clarify roles and responsibilities, and ensure necessary information is available for key decision-making meetings.

It is important to meet with senior colleagues in key agencies. Support from Directors and Heads of Services in CSC and NHS can help establish multi-agency meetings to discuss and agree the remit of the work, how it links with existing services, recruitment of children and families, and clinical information sharing. Detailed planning about how to implement the work in the local context avoids duplication of service provision and optimises good working relationships.

Service developments and changes across agencies can be challenging. Time spent in building and maintaining multi-agency relationships and getting feedback about the work is essential.

At the start of the SUSI study, discussions were held with key stakeholders about how to develop the clinical offer to minimise the workload and streamline requests to practitioners in other agencies. Much as clinical and research initiatives, and ultimately better services for children and families, may be welcomed, any change inevitably places additional demands on services.

Social workers, amongst other professionals, were relieved that at a time when few clinical resources are available, a focused assessment and intervention would be offered early.

Team meetings and service days were attended for colleagues across health and social care. In particular for teams with statutory involvement with families, it was important to outline the aims and processes of the work in some detail, e.g. familiarising staff with written information and clarifying the parameters of the SUSI study where there were research ethical requirements. There was an opportunity to discuss and underline the importance of working together to engage parents who may feel reluctant and anxious to engage. These meetings provided a useful opportunity to clarify SUSI aims and objectives, and to underline the multi-agency shared agreement and responsibility for the children, some of whom were already identified as being at risk. Colleagues, including social workers, thought about how the work would be carried out and were encouraged to give feedback as the study progressed. Staff appreciated having succinct and clear information about the purpose and aim of the work and this set a helpful basis for more collegiate work.

Regular meetings were held to provide updates, share experiences and discuss current issues identified in the SUSI work, such as gaining consent, legal interface and requests for court reports, and the importance of attending feedback meetings.

In the sections below, the key stakeholder groups have been identified, and the specific teams that were engaged with. Other localities may be configured differently so communication pathways could be adapted accordingly.

Strong partnership working is central to good, effective service delivery. Economic and targeted use of resources is important so that every opportunity is taken to share service aims, objectives, and to develop ways of working together.

Children's Social Care (CSC) department

Colleagues in CSC have a wide range of roles that include:

- Independent Reviewing Officers (IROs)
- adoption social workers
- fostering social workers
- Child Protection (CP) chair
- children's social workers in the care section, safeguarding and family support teams
- CSC administrative teams
- CSC legal team.

It was necessary to meet the CSC Director and heads of service promptly to define the clinical project offer and mutual areas of interest and benefit. The Director of the local CSC was a joint applicant for the funding, so the ownership of the work was held at a strategic level. At this early stage, the easiest way to access information was agreed; for example, CSC administration provided weekly lists of children who were eligible for the project. In the project's borough, these were children newly looked after or new to a CP plan, and the name of their current social worker. The meetings with heads of services and individual teams provided an opportunity to find creative solutions to develop clinical and information sharing pathways that were more robust and sensitive than existing working practice. In particular we wanted to achieve less burdensome ways of communicating and agree the best ways of working together. Each team had a different emphasis and role to fulfil, so it was important to understand this and shape communication and service delivery accordingly.

There are specific timescales for core group meetings and reports for conferences when children are on a CP plan. As part of the SUSI protocol, the dates set for CP meetings were requested so that assessments could be completed within these timescales, and the assessment feedback discussed and agreed with parents. Finalised assessment reports were sent to parents, CP chairs and social workers before the scheduled meetings.

A similar process for looked after children review meetings chaired by IROs was also agreed. While this puts pressure on a clinical team in terms of assessment completion and deadlines for written reports, it was invaluable to ensure that up-to-date information was available for key decision-making meetings. Therefore, the social, emotional and mental health needs of both the child and their parents/primary caregivers were considered at these meetings. As well as the CSC deadlines, SUSI clinicians required the dates of Initial Health Assessments (IHA) from Child Health so that the following information could be made available to the SUSI therapists:

- clinical information
- views on a child's social–emotional needs
- indication of any further assessments needed (neurodevelopmental, speech and language assessments)
- gaps in information
- clinical urgency.

The aim was to support the CSC team with their care plans for children and families.

Where there are plans for adoption, the CSC Adoption/Permanence teams require information from the SUSI assessment to be collated at an early stage to minimise delay in the adoption process. Adoption teams also have specific timescales. They need to ensure that clinical information about the child, who may have been assessed and treated while in care, can be shared with adoptive parents. CSC legal teams require clarity about timescales and often request that reports be shared with courts as part of care proceedings (see consent in the clinical governance section later in this chapter).

This knowledge of the various timelines, and sharing information accordingly, is vital in a project or clinical service context. It helps to ensure that recommendations from the SUSI assessments can be used to keep the focus on the child at a stressful and demanding time for families. Clinical practice shows that adults'/parents' needs can sometimes overshadow or compete with the child's social-emotional development needs. It is not unusual at these important times of decision-making that the clinical urgency for developmental opportunities for the child is eclipsed. Timely, succinct reports and recommendations from the SUSI assessments and intervention give the parents and statutory decision makers a 'view of the child' and their needs. From professionals' feedback, it is clear that they valued having reports that specifically focused on the child's presentation, developmental needs and capacity within the child/parent relationship. This can become a point of tension between agencies and this dynamic will be explored further in later chapters.

Adult Mental Health (AMH)

Regular links with key service members in a large service like AMH are important to:

- share areas of learning and clinical interest
- keep under review the possibility of joint service initiatives.

Generally, Child and Adolescent Mental Health Services (CAMHS) and AMH are very separate agencies with little overlap. This is unfortunate and, in many ways, uneconomic as a better sharing of information, clinical intelligence and governance can lead to better service provision. Given our populations of parents and under 5s, it is particularly important to have links with Perinatal and Parental Mental Health (PMH) services. The clinical team was fortunate to have an established PMH team in the borough that agreed to be part of the SUSI project and support the recruitment of families. The manager of this team became a member of the SUSI multi-agency steering group. SUSI staff met with the PMH staff on an individual basis and joined some team meetings to better understand the team's aims and clinical practice. Together they could discuss the SUSI approach and any concerns or questions about introducing a new element to their service offer.

The preparation time spent with PMH colleagues clarified ways of working, expectations on staff and families, and developed practical resources, such as the introductory letter to families explaining the SUSI work. Literature relating to young children's emotional/developmental needs was shared and historical case examples were discussed to consider the model's relevance to their families. This was especially pertinent as there can be a mismatch between how well the parent is progressing, i.e. the parents may be much better since the initial referral to PMH/AMH, and how the parent can meet the child's emotional needs and address established relationship patterns. This is complicated further when the SUSI assessment may highlight cause for concern about the child's development, a view not shared by other agencies, especially in the absence of obvious behavioural difficulties in the child. It can be painful to see that a parent's efforts and positive intentions for their child are not having the impact necessary to support the child's social–emotional development. We empathise with and need to work together to support parents, many of whom struggle day to day with the impact from an emotionally impoverished childhood themselves, current social adversity (domestic abuse, poor housing, isolation) and poverty.

Regular communication between staff in SUSI and PMH was needed to support cohesive care planning to address the child's and parent's emotional and mental health presentations. SUSI staff joined PMH scheduled meetings to:

1. cross check referrals or potential participants
2. discuss how each team's clinical focus and intervention complemented and supported work with specific families
3. agree joint home visiting and assessment feedback sessions.

There were times when a parent's disturbance became more apparent during the SUSI intervention, e.g. parents feeling suicidal, expressing a wish to harm the infant, evidence of more obsessive or psychotic symptomology. This had to be addressed urgently with robust plans to meet both the individual parent's needs and the child's needs with a multi-agency approach.

Communication with AMH colleagues provided updates on the project's progress and encouraged staff to contact us with ideas so that we could work as closely as possible. However, this highlighted gaps between these services and a need for stronger links to help raise awareness of the child's needs when their parent has a significant mental health difficulty.

Child Health

Community paediatricians play an essential role with looked after children (LAC) and children on a child protection (CP) plan. The interface between physical and social-emotional development and their impact and influences on each other is widely acknowledged (Avan, Richter, Ramchandani, Norris & Stein, 2010; Piek, Barrett, Smith, Rigoli & Gasson, 2010) so this work lends itself to close links and in many cases joint working.

The mainstream LAC CAMHS team had a close working relationship with the Child Health team who were closely involved in both the pilot screening project as well as in the SUSI study. In addition to the paediatricians, we met with Child Health nurses, speech and language therapists, and occupational therapists, as many of the children had complex developmental presentations. In some cases, parents had a strong belief that a 'diagnosis' would explain all of the presenting difficulties even when there were strong indicators that there was an emotional or relational contribution to the overall presentation.

Clarity with parents about information sharing with Child Health from an early stage, and about SUSI's role and practice, helped support the close clinical monitoring and liaison that was needed during the work with children and families. For example, parents recruited to SUSI were asked if they would agree to relevant clinical information being shared with Child Health. If during the course of our assessment a developmental need was identified, it was discussed with parents and their consent was gained to refer to Child Health for specific developmental assessments. This ensured the most effective care plan, with reviews for children sometimes taking place jointly with SUSI and Child Health staff.

Children's Centres and Early Help

Children's Centres are a great resource in terms of their knowledge of local families and in providing a range of services for children and families in accessible family-friendly premises. However, as discussed above, introducing a new way of working and any assumed similarity or difference to other interventions needs careful setting up, joint discussion and planning. While there are many interventions targeting parents and children, the focus on the child may be limited as few specifically assess the child's social-emotional needs (NSPCC, 2016; National Institute for Health and

Care Excellence, 2012). It is important to revisit normal child development and be able to identify difficulties in the child that do not routinely raise anxiety in the staff, e.g. the withdrawn, undemanding baby who looks 'fine' but already has adapted to the parent's need to be quiet and compliant, or the toddler who may seemingly be 'playing happily' on the floor but on close observation is not engaged in meaningful play but distracted and hypervigilant. Revisiting these clinical examples in the context of also having empathy for the often distressed parent, helped demonstrate the value of introducing a new assessment.

As the SUSI project recruited families, the Children's Centres were keen to support work happening within them and to join with facilitating more individual family bespoke 'packages' (for example, by identifying rooms and facilitating meetings in the Centres). Parents who are isolated and anxious, and who struggle to leave the house, may need help to attend a Children's Centre to complete the assessment and intervention. Conversely, sometimes parents need to be seen initially at home to minimise the possibility of them becoming distracted by the busy life at the Children's Centre.

Voluntary sector

Each locality is different but it is a great shame that many communities have lost access to important and valuable voluntary services, which often provide creative and flexible groups to families. Where they do exist it is important to include them in discussions to ensure that services are well used. There may be a concern that we are all 'competing' for the same families, especially when funding is not secure. While services are seeing the same families, the service provided by SUSI was very specific and focused on the child and the parent–child relationship. Although the SUSI work complemented other services and provided information about the child's social–emotional needs, regular communication was needed to help address different perspectives of the child's and parent's needs across the network (described further in Chapter 8). In the SUSI study, many complex cases were managed successfully with close collaboration with voluntary agencies.

Primary Care

Direct contact with GPs took place with routine letters following assessment, at review time-points and at the end of the intervention. There was also close involvement when parents had specific health problems, e.g. neurological conditions, mental health difficulties, cancer, or relationship stressors such as domestic violence.

There were ongoing links with Health Visitors (HV) and Family Nurse Partnership (FNP) practitioners with families on CP plans. Health Visitors joined us in consent meetings with families where they had particular concerns and established relationships with the parents. These professionals continued to be involved and joined the assessment and intervention feedback meetings with the parent's agreement where all agreed this to be beneficial. Where FNP nurses were working with families known to SUSI, we met to share perspectives and findings. FNPs and HVs welcomed the focus on the child's individual social-emotional development and thinking about the emotional quality of the relationship between the parent and the child.

SUSI assessment reports, and the individualised 'Activity templates' (see Chapter 5) created for parents, were often used by HVs and other professionals in their ongoing work with parents and children. These were always shared with the parents' expressed agreement.

CAMHS

Senior staff within the South London and Maudsley (SLAM) NHS Trust were well-informed of the work and involved in discussions in the planning stage, with the study proposal being supported by the Service Director. This work has an implication for already burdened CAMHS teams because, when a group is targeted, there is a very high possibility that more clinical need will be identified and more referrals made to existing CAMHS services. For looked after children specifically, it was advantageous that the work was developed as part of an existing and established LAC CAMHS team so referrals could go to this team at the end of the study if needed.

Overall few very young children are being referred to CAMHS teams. However, occasionally for children with particular behavioural or risk issues (self-harm, animal cruelty), the child known to SUSI may also have been referred to the LAC CAMHS. In these cases, the SUSI assessment was completed as it was more comprehensive and sensitive to the developmental stages of the child and the parent–child relationship. Depending on the assessment recommendations, care status and age of the child (near to 5) and/or the entrenched nature of the difficulties, joint work with CAMHS can be indicated at times.

Another point of contact with existing generic CAMHS can be when older siblings are referred to their teams while the younger children are identified for SUSI. Again good practice, liaison and sensitive appointment planning is needed.

Education

The Early Years Foundations Stage (EYFS) sets standards for the development, care and learning of children from birth to 5 years old. Liaison with colleagues in the EYFS took place throughout the assessment and intervention, with the agreement of parents and professionals where they held parental responsibility (PR).

Children seen in the clinical services and studies attended a variety of early years providers, e.g. nurseries, pre-schools and childminders. Contact with their key workers does provide invaluable insight and information for the assessment, giving a perspective on how the child is functioning and relating to adults and children when separate from their primary caregiver.

In the assessment phase, the child's key worker is asked to complete an Ages and Stages Questionnaire: Social-Emotional (ASQ:SE). It is also useful to have a direct discussion to unpick a child's presentation, especially where the key worker may have observed a behaviour or response from the child that is hard to understand or articulate. These details add to a developing and holistic picture of the child's needs and give insight into how they may require support going forwards. In addition, a sense is gained of how the child's internal model is influencing their capacity to trust others and establish and maintain wider relationships. One of the ASQ:SE questions in the older age band asks if the child can name a friend. It is not uncommon for the worker (or parent) to answer 'No' to this with a corresponding deep sense of sadness. Some of the children are so overwhelmed by trying to manage their own emotional states that they are unable to reach out and share enjoyment with their peers. Indeed for some children the usual conflicts that arise between peers are unmanageable and lead to emotional withdrawal, distress and/or outbursts of aggression.

One outcome following the assessment feedback can be the creation of an individualised 'Activity Template' for the parents, and these are often shared (with some adaptations as appropriate) with early years education workers. The Activity Template gives brief practical ideas on how to engage a child and extend their social interaction and/or play, with a particular focus on the adult's support for the child's emotional states. Ways that this can be approached by the worker are suggested and discussed along with the parent's involvement. (Individualised Activity templates can be also be created by downloading them from www.susiweb.co.uk.)

Contact with the early years providers informs existing and new networks as a child moves to the next stage of their education. The SUSI approach involves key workers in review/network meetings as much as possible. Joint discussions lead to a better insight into the child and family, to chart progress, and to find a shared language to consider their ongoing needs.

Establishing working practices

Senior working group

A multi-agency senior group, for example a steering group, that meets regularly (approximately two to three times a year) is a helpful, independent and invaluable reference point for any service. It is important that the membership reflects the community stakeholders (CSC, Legal, AMH, CAMHS, Child Health) and that it can act as a 'critical friend' to the work. The membership is strengthened if there can also be external representation, particularly from academic departments which have experience and expertise in research, service evaluation and implementation of clinical work. It is also helpful to include therapists who have expertise in the clinical area. The SUSI steering group had representatives from all of the above.

Gathering a 'team' with different viewpoints can add to the challenges. However, it also helps a great deal because it can:

- offer an opportunity to discuss different views and tensions between academics and therapists about clinical work in the community, leading to creative solutions
- offer clear time-points when the team have to present qualitative and quantitative data on clinical service provision and research data if it is within a new clinical service or research study. Discussion of this data guides service adaptations and provision
- add an external lens and strengthen the governance of the clinical work

- help the team keep in touch with other developments in the community and in other localities
- offer support and constructive feedback to the clinical team
- help the clinical team translate research findings into clinical practice.

An additional advantage is that busy clinical teams often feel neglected, or only thought about when data needs to be collected, or when they get reminders about administrative tasks. A steering group gives the wider clinical team the experience of their work being taken seriously, and being thought about. Feedback and views from the steering group were welcomed in the SUSI team.

Local pathways and clinical governance

On the basis of earlier planning meetings with partner agencies and knowledge of running a multi-disciplinary team (MDT) that works closely with other agencies, a map was made of how to work together. There was an awareness that this had to be kept under constant review because things change rapidly in services. When the SUSI project began, there was a whole service transformation in CSC which meant a reconsideration of how best to implement the SUSI model in the borough.

Operational policies, guidelines, screening protocols and specific forms for the clinical files were developed prior to staff coming into post and finalised as the recruitment of children and families began. These included:

- home visiting procedures
- risk assessment forms
- demographic data collection
- communication pathways of potential participants by partner agencies
- development of introduction letters to participants
- operational delivery of screening
- the outline of the intervention handbook.

As part of the NHS, the SUSI team adhered to the Trust's safeguarding policy, complaints procedures and guidelines for clinical responsibility. Local and national working guidance was included in the generic Trust induction. However, staff were also provided with a local SUSI induction to agree the specific application of wider guidance and reporting lines. This was reviewed throughout the work in the team.

As the SUSI model was trialled in a feasibility study, both patient information leaflets and consent sheets were developed. In the study design phase these were shared with CSC teams (safeguarding, care, adoption and fostering) and the PMH team so they were aware of the specifics of the process and were familiar with what the families would be asked at the point of consent. The possibilities of the SUSI work were discussed, as well as the limitations. This information was also shared with CP Chairs and IROs. Within the study context, the different NHS ethical research requirements specific to this study needed to be clarified with colleagues, particularly in terms of consent and information sharing and how it differed from a clinical service.

Both written information and visual materials that include service descriptions and inter-agency communication need to be available to families so they are fully informed of the process from the beginning. This provides not only clarity about what service is being offered, and what is required from the family, but is also another opportunity to discuss with the family any anxieties or reservations they may have about embarking on this work. Experience showed that these conversations resulted in better engagement from the families as they felt more involved in the consent process.

Consent deserves a specific mention as it was a key point that needed clarifying at the recruitment stage of the process and later when there were requests to share information (assessment and/or intervention reports) with the courts if a family moved from CP to care proceedings. For the purpose of the research we were clear that consent to information sharing had to be given by the parents. However, before they could join the study, they had to consent to assessment and intervention reports being shared with their allocated social worker and CP Chair IRO respectively. There was considerable discussion with Southwark Legal and the Research Ethics committee to clarify these issues.

In terms of recruitment in the research study, it was necessary to approach the families independently of other agencies to let them know about the work and to make an appointment with them to discuss the detail of the SUSI assessment and consent procedure. Attempts were made to meet them before or after a scheduled meeting at CSC but this could be problematic as the meetings were liable to cancellation, or the family did not attend. This level of unpredictability is not unusual with families who are involved with statutory services. As many families found organisation and planning difficult, trying to set up a separate meeting with them added another stage and an additional challenge to the meeting taking place.

The progress and stages of families' involvement was monitored in SUSI weekly team meetings, as well as individual staff supervision. This helped to ensure that the study process could be adhered to while not compromising the clinical integrity of work with the children and families. Both individual and group supervision for clinical staff is described in Chapter 7.

Service delivery monitoring and audit/evaluation

To ensure clinical quality, services need to build in a monitoring and evaluation cycle. This is central to ensuring clinical governance. The World Health Organization divides clinical quality into four aspects:

1. professional performance (technical quality)
2. resource use (efficiency)
3. risk management (the risk of injury or illness associated with the service provided)
4. patients' satisfaction with the service provided.

For the NHS, high quality clinical care is an integral commitment and is at the heart of everyday practice. In setting up a new service, it is important to apply methods of continuous quality improvements. We stressed the need for a systems-wide approach, i.e. partner agencies being fully included in the planning and implementation of any new service initiative. From a platform of strong multi-agency working and shared philosophy it is possible to:

- build and develop a strong leadership and teamwork
- have a clear focus on children and families
- develop robust data collection and data systems.

Clinical work can then be reviewed and evaluated to ensure clinical and economic effectiveness.

The measures used in SUSI are all reliable as well as being deliverable in a community setting. Some have online training, e.g. Keys to Interactive Parenting Scale (KIPS), and can be administered to a mixed population. The KIPS can also be used as an outcome measure so changes in the parent–child relationship can be assessed at set time periods to measure the impact of intervention from time-points one and two. In conjunction with clinical assessment and socio-demographic information, this provides a solid basis on which to monitor and evaluate a service. The accuracy, completeness and analysis of this core clinical data not only enhances delivery of SUSI but has the added advantage of better service planning and administration. The measures can be added to but it is strongly recommended that the combination of measures focusing on the child, the parent–child relationship and the parent's well-being remain at the core of further SUSI initiatives.

Mechanisms for collecting feedback from children/families and professional groups greatly enhance services. This information can be used to shape the service and is sensitive to any local or borough-specific changes that may indicate a shift in practice in one agency. Indeed with a good basic system and a multifaceted strategy, it is possible for the multi-agency group to compare activity trends for the SUSI clinical group from one year to the next, e.g.:

- increase/decrease in referrals
- more children staying on or coming off CP plans sooner
- increased or reduced numbers coming into care
- more safeguarding referrals.

Experience from the project showed that the sharing of service evaluation information across agencies, with more transparent lines of responsibility and clarity of roles, facilitated joint working between services, e.g. CAMHS and Child Health, and CAMHS and CSC. Strong individual and group supervision should be used to promote professional development, and to identify and deal with any performance issues early on. With regular monitoring of the data, any problems with service delivery and organisation can be tackled.

The challenges of multi-agency work are often written about: anxieties about sharing practice, feelings of vulnerabilities, guilt about what has and has not been done. However, a multi-agency commitment and endeavour is an opportunity to enthuse and inspire. It holds the possibility of supporting individual staff in their work (social work with high risk families often feels like a lonely and frightening task); what before might have felt like increasing workload or demand can become a shared task. This collegiate and transparent practice, if supported, has the added benefit of allowing economic use of resources and offering a less fragmented experience to children and families.

Selection and training of staff

Significant time is rightly given to the planning of a service and its clinical rationale. However, the recruitment process for staff is a complicated one but worth investing in heavily. It is important that senior staff think very carefully about the clinical task, the population they are working with and the qualities as well as the qualifications that are needed for a post. Job descriptions need to be written carefully and while it is recognised that most services have standard job descriptions, it is possible to use the job purpose section to identify key elements of the job in hand. If possible, negotiate with your local Human Resources department to see if there are other aspects of the job description you can add to or expand on. Attention to detail in a job advertisement helps attract candidates who are genuinely interested in this area of work.

In any given clinical area, recruitment should not exclude candidates who have a good aptitude for the work but may have limited experience. Some clinicians choose to undertake a period of personal therapy in order to help manage their own responses to certain difficult situations which lead to a loss of their necessary objectivity. When recruiting for an under 5s team, it is helpful to have team members with mixed experience. Some members may have worked in AMH, neurodevelopmental services or adolescent teams. It may be more difficult to recruit CAMHS staff with clinical experience of work with under 5s and their parents. Therefore, specific training for staff regarding the SUSI model and infant mental health is needed.

The interview process is strengthened if potential candidates are tested in a variety of ways, e.g. giving observational feedback on a parent–child interaction, a group task, a written task in addition to individual interview. This gives the recruiting team a good sense of the capability and flexibility of applicants, and their interest and willingness to be open to different ways of working. It is important to identify applicants' strengths and limitations so that supervision and further training can be given. All staff will have direct contact with the families and need to demonstrate high quality communication and interpersonal skills.

Trust NHS induction offers staff knowledge of the wider context and offers a broad range of mandatory training. There is further specific training for staff in the SUSI assessment and intervention model, described in more detail in Chapter 9. A brief description of the training programme is outlined below.

TRAINING FOR THE CLINICAL AND RESEARCH STAFF WITHIN THE SUSI STUDY TEAM

1. training in infant and young children's developmental stages, social–emotional development and mental health presentations, parent–child attachment and relationship development for typical and maladaptive/abusive relationship patterns
2. training in recruitment and engagement of children and families
3. history-taking and use of specific child and parent–child measures in the initial clinical assessment and reviews, e.g. delivery of ASQ:SE, KIPS, Denver II (see Chapter 4 for more detail)
4. how to carry out the assessment in variety of contexts
5. report writing: format, style
6. liaison with and feedback of assessment to the family and network
7. delivery of the intervention
8. delivery of review assessments and associated clinical and network liaison
9. training and refinement of systems for the specific team setting
10. supervision structure to establish reflective space
11. team review systems for referrals and case allocation
12. systems for recording and safe-keeping of clinical and audit/outcomes data
13. access to SUSI model resources.

Group training of staff helps to develop team identity and cohesion of clinical aims. This helps to ensure adherence to the fidelity of the model.

4 Assessment of the child's social-emotional development and child-parent relationship

The assessments seemed really helpful and the families' feedback was that they found the staff and process very thoughtful - it helped them think about their issues in a different way and provided something tangible for them to work with.

PARENTAL MENTAL HEALTH WORKER

It was interesting to see how some subtle issues were observed early on about attachment and developmental issues for babies.

SOCIAL WORKER

A number of policy and review papers have been published recently by leading charity organisations, academic institutions and cross-party working groups. They highlight the impact that early childhood adversity has on an individual's development, health and well-being into adulthood (Building Great Britons, 2015; NSPCC, 2016; PIP UK, 2019).

Particular environmental risk factors (domestic abuse, parental mental health, prenatal stress and poverty) have been identified as potentially having the most detrimental impact on children, especially babies and very young children, whose development in the first two years is known to be especially sensitive to input from their social environment.

The quality of caregiving from a parent is known to be the primary source of support in establishing a child's sense of security and other aspects of their development. This caregiving mediates the effects of stress arising from early adversity. Therefore, attention has turned to the essential role of parent–child interaction and relationships in promoting a child's welfare. Understanding how stressors on the family may impact on the parent-child relationship has been highlighted as a necessary and core aspect of assessments with high-risk populations, and has become part of recommendations and guidance from experts in the field.

The box below summarises key recommendations from National Institute for Health and Care Excellence (NICE) and Social Care Institute for Excellence (SCIE) guidance and expert reports relating to under 5s' populations and those with specific vulnerabilities.

- NICE Early Years report (2012) refers to the evidence that a strong foundation of social-emotional well-being plays an important role in later educational and health outcomes. It recommends that 'targeted support (should be available) to those most in need'.
- Joint SCIE and NICE guidance for looked after children (2010) states that all under 5s should receive a CAMHS screening and timely intervention by a specialist child mental health practitioner.
- The Building Great Britons paper (All Party Parliamentary Group for Conception to Age 2, 2015) recommends that 'families involved with social care should have a routine assessment of parent-child interaction'.
- NICE (2017) produced the Child Abuse and Neglect guidance, recommending that interventions for under 5s should be attachment based. The aim is to improve caregivers' understanding of their child's cues and behaviours and to be responsive and nurturing to their child's needs and emotions.

Background

This assessment model is designed to explore and identify a child's social-emotional capacity and development in the framework of their relationship(s) with primary caregivers and attachment figures. It has been used successfully in community clinical trials and community services with vulnerable families with children and parents whose relationships have had diverse histories and starting points.

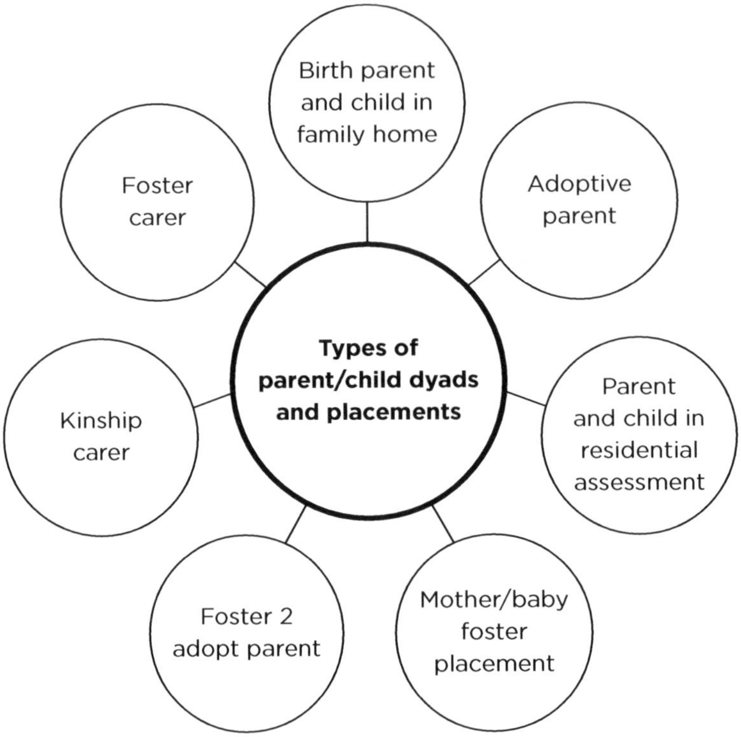

Figure 4.1 The different parent-child dyads that have been seen within this assessment model

Infant mental health and early years' assessments usually take place in the family home, as recommended by practitioners and experts in the field (Boris, Fueyo & Zeanah, 1997; Lieberman & Van Horn, 2008). The SUSI assessment followed this approach in general, but also gave options to the families about where to meet. For a significant number who were living in poor housing and cramped conditions, they opted to come to Children's Centres, nursery settings or the community CAMHS base (in a local health centre).

Many of the babies and children were living with their parents in the family home and had experienced no major separations from their primary caregiver(s). Other parents and children had formed new relationships after the child-birth parent relationship was disrupted due to health, social or risk factors. The time varied at which we began to engage with the family and learn about the babies'/children's needs and development across a

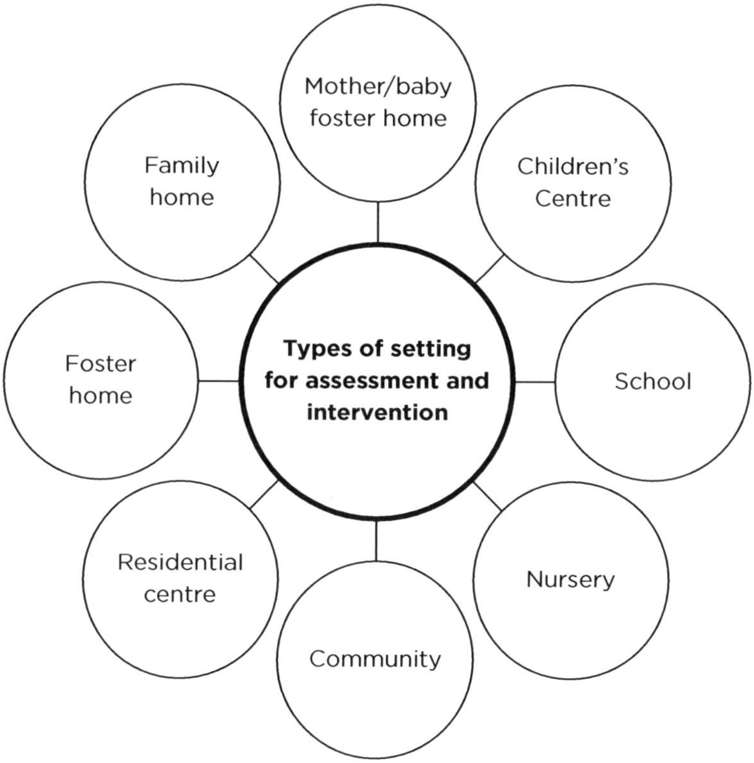

Figure 4.2 The different types of locations used to deliver the assessment

0–4-year age span. It was dictated to by the circumstances that brought the families into contact with health and/or social services. Therefore, a model was needed that could focus on the central issues affecting the parent-children dyad but which could adapt to the diversity of contexts and types of families.

The clinical formulation derived from the assessment was broad based. There was a need to be thorough in exploring the many contributing factors to the children's presentation, remembering that these early years are a time of rapid change with both strengths and potential blocks constantly emerging along the children and parent's pathway together. The focus on the relationship includes other important aspects of child-parent relationships such as parental involvement, communication, shared experience and enjoyment. The specific focus on the children's individual developmental history and current skills crosses all developmental domains.

There is a continuous two-way influence between the emotional world of a young child and their capacity to grow and develop socially, physically and cognitively. At one extreme we know that a child can literally fail to grow and gain weight when in an emotionally impoverished and neglectful environment. This dynamic may also show in more subtle manifestations of temporarily being un-coordinated and physically unregulated when in a distressed state, giving a mind–body perspective to the commonly used phrase about 'feeling wobbly' (Van der Kolk, 2015).

There are many helpful descriptions in the research and clinical literature of how to approach and understand the experience of a child as well as a parent, and reflections on how these meet in the unique match between the pair (Stern, 1995). We will return to the other important relationships that both child and parent(s) have, but in the first instance will focus on the primary dyadic relationship with the adult(s) who provides the majority of their everyday care.

The rationale for a detailed focus on the child and their experience of the primary relationship is that it is essential to understand its complexity. However, this can be hard to extract for several reasons at this stage of their life. The children are often preverbal or have very limited communication apart from their physical or emotional behaviours and responses. Therefore the parent/carer is looked to, to describe their experiences and perspective. This may be causing them a great deal of concern or distress in itself, or conversely they may be out of touch with the concerns that others are expressing. While taking care to hear the parent's views and feelings and support them, it can be hard sometimes to have a robust focus on the child. An Independent Reviewing Officer (IRO) previously described that an assessment had given 'a voice to the child'. The SUSI model includes a range of clinical approaches and standardised measures which together try to articulate both children's and parents' experiences.

As the collective methods join to make up the final formulation, the next section will describe the core components of the assessment, incorporating clinical examples. The use of specific standardised measures and clinical observations are included in the descriptions of assessment and in case studies. (Note that the case studies are composite examples based on casework; they have been significantly modified to preserve anonymity.)

The practical process of assessment

Figure 4.3 on the next page outlines the main stages of the assessment process trialled in the research project and since delivered in a community clinical service. We will go on to explain how these stages are put into practice and made relevant to different contexts. (The approach has to be tailored to integrate into a range of settings when delivered elsewhere.)

The assessment has been outlined as a combination of both standardised measures and clinical observations and discussion. Each informs the other to gather a detailed profile of the child and the parent(s), and the child's relationship in any given social and cultural context. The conversations with parents are both a source of information and an important part of relationship-building. Descriptions are given below of the standardised measures used in SUSI and our clinical service as these will then be referenced to help illustrate the practical application of the assessment process.

Assessment measures

PARENT-CHILD DYAD

Keys to Interactive Parenting Scale (KIPS; Comfort & Gordon, 2006; Comfort, Gordon & Naples, 2011)

KIPS is a reliable, evidence-based tool to effectively measure parenting behaviours. Twelve aspects of parenting (e.g. sensitivity of responses, physical interaction, involvement in child's activities, adapts strategies to child, etc.) were rated on a five-point scale, following a 10 minute observation of the parent/carer interacting with the child. The parenting behaviours are classified in one of these three domains:

1. building relationships
2. promoting learning
3. supporting confidence.

In the validation of the KIPS inter-rater reliability, coefficients were very high ranging from .90 to .96. The 12 KIPS subscales are averaged to form a single rating of positive parent-child interaction (α = .89). It has also been shown to have good face validity through focus groups, and good sensitivity shown through significant changes following a year of intervention. KIPS scores were also categorised as low quality interactions, moderate quality interactions or high quality interactions for comparison (Comfort, Gordon & Unger, 2006).

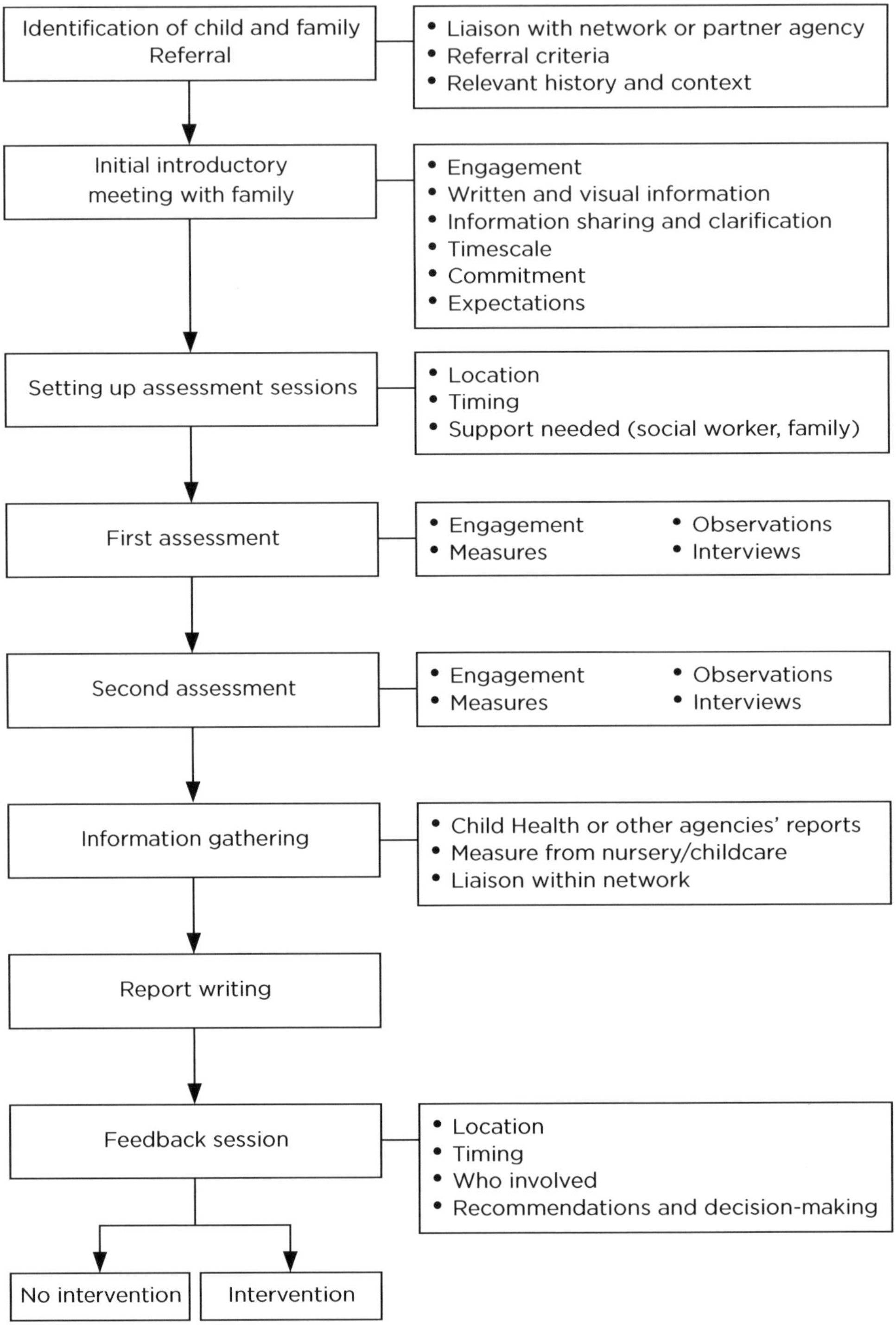

Figure 4.3 Flowchart of the assessment process

CHILD

The Ages and Stages Questionnaire Social-Emotional (ASQ:SE)
ASQ:SE (Squires, Bricker and Twombly, 2003; 2015) addresses the social and emotional behaviour of children aged from 2 to 65 months. There are seven behavioural areas of:

- self-regulation
- compliance
- communication
- adaptive
- autonomy
- affective functioning
- interaction with people.

These areas are addressed in separate questionnaires for children at six monthly age intervals, each taking about 15–20 minutes to complete in a semi-structured interview with the CAMHS practitioner. Test-retest reliability and inter-rater reliability have both been calculated at 94%. Criterion validity has been calculated to give a sensitivity rate of 78% and a specificity rate of 95%.

The Denver II (Frankenburg, Dodds, Archer, Shapiro & Bresnick, 1992)
This assesses four domains of child development:

- personal–social
- fine motor
- language
- gross motor.

The test is primarily based upon an examiner's direct observation of the child rather than parental report. The tests cover the age range from birth to 6 years. Based on the child's age, scores can either be 'normal', 'suspect' or 'untestable'. The Denver II has inter-rater and test-retest reliability of 0.99 ± 0.01 and 0.90 ± 0.12, respectively. Criterion validity has been calculated to give a low specificity rate (43%) but balanced with a high sensitivity rate (83%) (Glascoe et al., 1992).

Adverse Child Experiences (ACE; Bellis, Lowey, Leckenby, Hughes & Harrison, 2014)
An ACE score was calculated for each child based on information collected during the assessment. Scores of 4 or more indicate significant vulnerability for physical and mental health disorders later in life.

PARENT

Depression, Anxiety and Stress 21 Test (DASS 21, a shortened version of the DASS: Lovibond & Lovibond, 1995)

This is a questionnaire designed to measure the severity of a range of symptoms related to the negative emotional states of depression, anxiety and stress. The DASS is suitable for both adolescents and adults. The instrument is based on participant responses to 21 questions, relating to each of the three scales. This measure was only administered to birth parents in any study group. DASS has good overall reliability (a = .93). Henry and Crawford (2005) also reported subscales to be reliable measures of depression (a = .88), anxiety (a = .82), and stress (a = .90). Normative data were based on a large UK sample (N = 1,794) of 18- to 91-year olds.

Demographic information

This information was collected for all families, from a range of sources. Information about the child and family was routinely asked for during the two assessment sessions, e.g. pregnancy/birth history, any health or developmental concerns for the child, health (physical and mental) concerns for the parent and their education level. For families in the social care groups, where specific consent had been obtained, the team had access to background reports from Children's Social Care. Additional information was gathered from families throughout the course of their involvement with the assessment, intervention or reviews.

Practical delivery of assessment

As discussed in Chapter 2, an outreach targeted population approach was chosen in both the pilot and the SUSI projects. This meant that the offer of the assessment was made to all eligible families who fitted the criteria for inclusion. We did not wait for other professionals or agencies to make referrals to us. The reasons for this approach were due to challenges within our current systems of identifying early signs of distress or dysfunction in young babies/children. (The problem was compounded by there generally being limited knowledge and confidence in how to discuss the social-emotional needs of babies and young children with their parents.)

Consent

Within the SUSI study we carried out a consent visit with each family to discuss their involvement in the project. This included information on the structure and different stages of the work. Information was given to clarify how details were shared with the network, and this offered a chance for the family to ask any questions and seek clarification. This helped to allay some parents' anxiety who had specific worries, e.g. about whether they would be separated from their child during appointments. We could clarify how the meetings would work on a practical level for them. Often the family would bring another family member or key worker from the network.

While gaining consent is a necessary but time-consuming stage of any research project, it also has many advantages: it helps to make the proposed work more transparent, allowing detailed discussions about what this will entail for the family and how it fits with other parts of their network. This was especially important for parents who were experiencing worry or distrust in relationships with professionals or agencies, perhaps being on the edge of statutory or legal involvement in their lives. We could be clear about how our input could inform others' views, plans and the multi-agency support package. This resulted in some families declining involvement as they did not want their GP to be informed, or their social worker where there was CSC involvement to receive the assessment. Many mainstream community services have information leaflets to give to service users about their appointments, as we do within our clinical service. As the consent process involved a greater level of detail, it seemed a useful aspect of the initial engagement and may have contributed to the high level of retention at follow-up time-points. Similar resources to those developed for the research study could be used as a basis for service protocols and information leaflets for families in community teams.

Referral meetings

In a mainstream service with a more commonly used referral system, there may be a referral meeting, similar to the consent visit described above. A discussion can be held with the family about the process, and thought can be given to practical considerations of timing and location, and whether to include other relevant people in the appointments, in order to complete the assessment. In both clinical service and research settings, allocation of a practitioner to the family was made in a weekly team meeting. The allocation of the worker was based on the specific needs of the family, and where possible the therapist who conducted the initial referral meeting would be appointed. There is strong evidence that this continuity helped families to remain engaged with the work. This was especially important with families who were already under great strain.

The assessment was usually completed in two visits that took place in the preferred location of the parent. In the majority of cases, home visits were undertaken to complete all aspects of the assessment, but some families chose to attend the clinic or meet at a community location with which they were familiar. The assessment was also delivered in residential settings if the family was living there.

The assessment was completed with the primary caregiver, with fathers/secondary carers actively encouraged to take part and contribute to the assessment. As there were several variations in the caregiver–child dyad, the participants involved differed, for example when a child was looked after by a foster carer the assessment took place in the foster home with them and the child. In such cases, the birth parents were invited to meet separately to complete the ASQ:SE in a semi-structured interview, to discuss their views on their child's needs. Correspondingly, when birth parents were the primary caregiver in mother–baby foster placements, the foster carers were invited to contribute to the assessment. For children already in nursery, teachers also completed the standardised ASQ:SE questionnaires when parental permission was given.

Measures and interviews

The measures and interviews were delivered during the assessment visits in a flexible way that was sensitive to the needs of the child and family at the time. In some cases, the child needed an opportunity to 'warm' to the therapist before they were able to complete the Denver measure. In other cases, the parent needed time to feel comfortable and therefore the ASQ:SE or Denver would be completed first. Time was allowed for the parents to expand on specific questions asked in the child and adult measures. This was particularly important when administering the ASQ:SE and DASS questionnaires, as some parents were anxious about potential consequences if they admitted to difficulties. Other parents seemed unaware of specific behaviours and responses being of possible concern. When completing the DASS, the therapist would follow the lead of the parents, some of whom wished to talk in much more detail about their feelings and experiences.

The KIPS play observation was completed with the primary caregivers, and where available secondary carers. This allowed the team to view how the child interacted with different people. Prior to the observation, the parent was asked to spend 10 minutes playing and interacting with their child, with their own choice of activity, which could include talking or singing with babies and younger children.

When consent to video was given, the observation was recorded using a hand-held video camera. Where families did not wish to be recorded, two staff members would attend the session that included the timed parent-child observation to ensure observations were collected reliably. Immediately following the visit, the staff would rate the interaction observation so that the detail could be captured and agreement on the ratings could be reached while the observation was fresh in their minds.

In addition to the standardised measures, considerable time was allowed for conversations with the parents, together with informal observations of the child and the parent-child interaction. These complemented the information gathering that the measures sought and gave opportunities to explore some of the key issues or concerns that the parent raised when completing the measures. It also helped to inform the therapist's understanding of the many factors contributing to the child and family's experience. The unstructured time was an important part of the engagement process and was used to reflect on how to approach the feedback of the assessment to the parent(s).

The clinical assessment

The above section describes some key points of structure relating to how the assessment was delivered. The core clinical features of the assessment will now be explored, divided into the constructs of:

- the child-parent relationship
- the parent's views and representations
- the child's individual development.

Child-parent relationship

Informal clinical observations are a key aspect of understanding the current presentation of the child-parent relationship. They help to inform and reflect on the history of this with the parent. Time is needed to see how the parent and child relate to one another in unstructured moments, noting

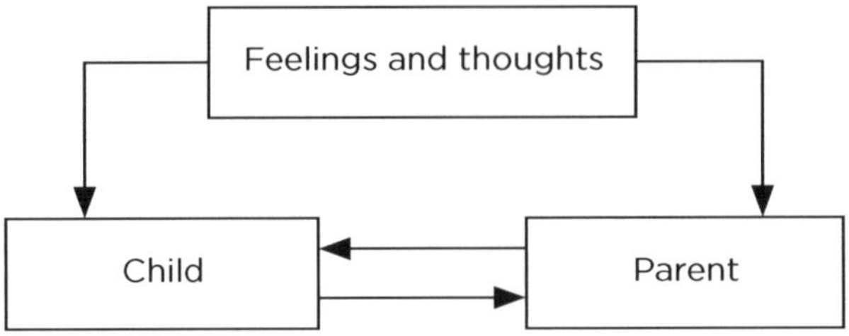

Figure 4.4 The 'to-and-fro' of the parent-child relationship

how variations between visits may be influenced by the family becoming more comfortable with the workers. Other factors could also include the presence or absence of other family members. The family may have been affected by particular stressors which occurred prior to a visit. For some families who experience chaotic lifestyles, it is not unusual for circumstances to change unpredictably. Any contrasts or similarities of the interaction patterns between these more naturalistic periods and that of the timed 'play' observation can be noted.

Reflections on how these different moments are experienced may be possible with the parent at the time. This will depend on the emotional state and insight of the parent, and to what degree thoughts and feelings are triggered at the time. For example, one parent described how moving from the more focused play time back to their normal interaction had brought to light how little time they would usually spend in any close interaction; and that their usual state of distance from each other was painful to reflect on.

Alongside the general points of reference above, the therapist observes specific responses of the parent to the child's expressions of general communication, or cues for emotional and practical support, and how the parent anticipates if the child requires particular input and interaction. This includes the presence or not of attachment-related behaviours when the activation of the child's attachment system could be expected. According to the age of the child, consideration is given to the stage of attachment development and the behavioural shifts that occur at key times across the early years (Zeanah, Berlin & Boris, 2011). We can observe what balance there is between attachment and exploratory behaviours on the child's part for those beyond infancy, and how each of these contrasting behaviours is responded to by the parent. Particular notice can be given to how any imbalance may be reinforced by the parent. Close attention is needed to observe whether there is an absence of communications or emotions from the child towards the parent, and what strategies the child uses to manage in the situation. The case study that follows illustrates these points.

CASE STUDY A

A was 9 months when we undertook our initial assessment. He was the first child of his parents who were busy professionals and both struggling with the adjustment to parenthood. A's mother expressed feelings of having made a terrible mistake, being a 'bad mother' and of having thoughts to harm him. There were difficulties at night-time with A finding it hard to settle to sleep. This created high levels of stress for all.

Other difficulties identified at assessment included: conflict at feeding times; A being overly independent; resistance to being picked up; poor eye contact. Observing mum and son together, the therapist was struck by how 'manic' their interactions were during play, when they would both become increasingly excitable and loud. There were no moments of calm face to face interaction. A did not look to his mum when he needed support and, when he became fretful, mum would sweep him up, rock him wildly and sing loudly. These features of their relationship were included sensitively in the feedback assessment which Mum accepted and felt understood by, and she and A's father expressed a wish for things to change and to have the support of the intervention. ●●●

By noting both the most common cycles of relating and any situation-specific ones (e.g. if another family member joins) we can build a sense of the relating styles and capacity of the parent and child to engage emotionally in reciprocal interaction or play. For example, we may observe that the parent is highly responsive when the interaction is going smoothly and the child's emotional state is calm or positive, but that their responsiveness and quality of engagement changes if the child needs more support from them, even at momentary signs of frustration or dysregulation. These times provide the chance to hear more about the parent's own emotional state and their expectations of the child. The latter may or may not be consistent with other descriptions or beliefs about the child that the parent has given. Equally if a child's observed responses to the parent or

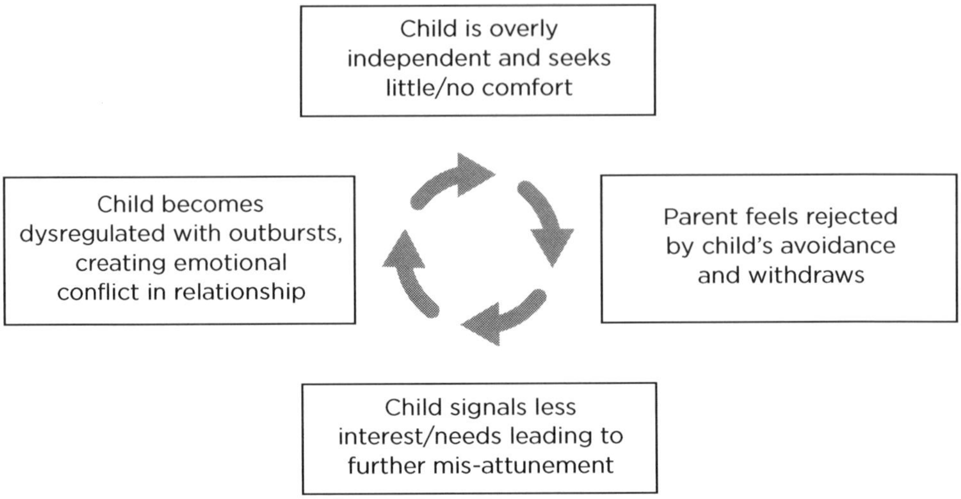

Figure 4.5 Cycles of interaction

therapist vary greatly from the parent's other narratives about the child, this needs to be noted and thought about further, e.g. a child is described as never approaching strangers but makes immediate demands on the therapist for comfort or help.

As described earlier, KIPS is used alongside the clinical observations to provide a reliable benchmark for parental behaviours towards the child across the three domains of:

- building relationships
- promoting learning
- supporting confidence.

With its emphasis on what observable actions the parent takes to promote their child's sense of emotional security, as well as cognitive, language and play development, it provides the opportunity to take a structured approach to rating how emotionally attuned and practically skilled the parent is in different aspects of parenting with an individual child. By rating 12 separate behaviours, it provides an opportunity to distinguish between different areas of specific strengths or limitation that the parent demonstrates. This can afford some balance in situations where there could be a tendency to give a generalised overview of the relationship.

CASE STUDY B

B was a 6-month-old baby girl who was living with an experienced and sensitive foster carer. She had previously been living with her mother for her first three months in a mother–baby foster placement which had come to an end. Since then she had regular contact with her mother several times a week.

B's foster carer did not have any concerns about her, and they seemed to enjoy quite active play where she bounced up and down, smiling, with her carer responding warmly. Initially, the therapist had thought the interaction was going well throughout. However, on reflection, we considered the moments in between the 'exciting' play, when she would look blank and be unresponsive to her carer, who in turn looked at a loss to know how to engage with her. She could also only fleetingly accept comfort before pulling away and trying to initiate more of the physical play again.

Through the feedback discussion, the different aspects of her presentation could be thought about some more, and the carer acknowledged that she experienced her as very changeable, and quite unreachable at times. The carer wanted to help her to relate and be more social in an ordinary and consistent way. We thought that this would support B's emotional security and in turn could also help her develop play and cognitive skills (with which she was showing some delay). ●●●

The expectation that the parent will interact or play with their child for a set time can be more or less challenging depending on how usual it is for them to engage like this in everyday life. The therapist provides reassurance and containment to the parent, reassuring them that the play or activity can be ordinary. They may discuss what the parent feels most comfortable with so that they take time to get the context right for themselves and their child. If the parent agrees, this process is videoed and can then be reviewed and rated with trained colleagues to gain other opinions (and to provide inter-rater reliability when follow-up KIPS are carried out for outcome purposes). Positive feedback on any aspects of an individual's parenting is important, as well as sensitively addressing areas of difficulty. The KIPS can provide helpful insights and contribute to these discussions.

Throughout the work in exploring the parent–child relationship, we need to be mindful and alert to observable risk behaviours, or mental state indicators, in both the parent and child, and within the parent–child relationship. Sometimes these can be fleeting signs – a gesture or expression – or there may be repeating cycles of interaction or behaviours. All should be noted and recorded and explored more, either directly with the parent or within reflective discussions in the team. We can also use our own emotional responses to distressing or disturbing interactions, or specific episodes in the visit, to reflect on further in case reviews and supervision to contribute to our understanding of the issues.

Parents and children may have established highly entrenched patterns of relating. These may be similar to descriptions of insecure attachment classifications, where the child's adaptive response to the parent's anxious or troubled state of mind results in them presenting with very emotional, disorganised or withdrawn behaviours (Cassidy, 1994). There may also be contradictory responses from the child, described as clinical disorders of attachment in toddlers (Lieberman & Van Horn, 2008). We need to be aware of the specific atypical parental responses outlined in the AMBIANCE classification model (Lyons-Ruth, Bronfman & Parsons, 1999). Among others, these include a parent interacting in a contradictory, frightening or care-seeking way with the child.

Patterns may be long established and become organised to match the parent's capacity for emotional regulation in the relationship. From an early age, the child becomes an active contributor to these cycles of relating if they have by necessity had to adapt to their caregiver's needs primarily. The influence from child to adult is seen particularly when a child moves from one primary caregiver to another and similar patterns can become organised with the new carer within days or weeks (Stovall-McClough & Dozier, 2004).

CASE STUDY C

At the time of the assessment, C was 2 years old and living with her mother and father in a residential assessment centre. The assessment from the unit, in part informed by the SUSI report, was negative for both parents and C was placed in foster care.

With her parents, C was presenting with significant emotional and behavioural difficulties including extreme outbursts of emotion, being unable to regulate herself or accept support to calm down and be comforted, followed by episodes of being emotionally withdrawn. In foster care, although some of the presenting behavioural difficulties quickly reduced, she continued to show extreme emotional responses to ordinary events/moments and would become very provocative.

The assessment highlighted that although she appeared 'close' to her foster carer (wanting to engage in sharing, being upset when separated, having hugs and cuddles), there were many times that she did not seek or accept comfort when she needed her carer's support the most. The intervention therefore focused on addressing specific interactions so these core emotional needs could be met. ●●●

The parent's views and representations

When talking with a parent, we need to listen to their concerns and views so that they feel understood, and so that they understand we are committed to them throughout the uncertainty, anger, distress or confusion they may be experiencing. During these initial discussions we take note of the way that the parent thinks and reflects on their own and their child's emotions and actions. The detail and coherence of their narratives will help us to be sensitive to the underlying anxieties and blocks that influence their capacity to explore and think about different aspects of their own and their child's life (Slade, Grienenberger, Bernbach, Levy & Locker, 2005).

Parents are able to share information with us at different paces. Some parents use the assessment to think further about related memories or experiences, whether recent or from their childhood history. These may have been on their mind or triggered by some of the questions and discussions about the relationship with their child. Other parents will want to share current stressors, especially if these are directly impacting on their daily lives and causing high levels of stress, e.g. inadequate housing, immigration status, threats from or conflicts with an adult partner. Some parents are not ready to share much of their personal views or experiences at this stage, and all of these variations need the therapist to show sensitivity and respect.

CASE STUDY D

D was a 4-year-old boy who had a diagnosis of Autistic Spectrum Disorder (ASD). D's mum had recently left D's dad due to domestic abuse and was in temporary accommodation. Her immigration status limited her employment opportunities and most of her family lived outside the UK. She had been referred to an ASD support group which she attended. She spoke of finding it useful but emotionally hard as most parents attending were couples. She had used the assessment sessions in part to communicate the significant stress, loss and everyday challenges she was experiencing.

The assessment had also highlighted the relationship patterns that the mum and son were struggling with. In the intervention, she expressed a wish and commitment to understand more about D's emotional and social needs and their specific relationship. ●●●

CASE STUDY E

Child E's family were experiencing a great deal of stress from many sources and her mother was supported well through Parental Mental Health (PMH) to manage her own emotional distress. The family's immigration status meant they had no access to public funds.

Child E was around 3 years old at the time of assessment. In the preceding months an accident had hurt E, for which E's mother felt responsible and extremely guilty. Being able to discuss these worries with a separate PMH worker allowed her to spend the sessions focusing on her relationship with E. This freed her up from the guilt to make changes to her responses to and relationship with her daughter who was presenting with complex emotional and behavioural difficulties. ●●●

Whether linked or not through identification to themselves or other significant figures in their life, parents may give negative or distorted attributions to their child. These were described by Selma Fraiberg in the well-known concept of 'ghosts in the nursery' (Fraiberg, Adelson & Shapiro, 1975). As these identifications may be longstanding and strongly held beliefs, they should be approached with care and noted in terms of what can be observed as having a direct impact on the cycles of interaction between parent and child. Gentle questions and comments can be introduced to see if the parent can respond to the therapist's attempt to explore this further. The parent's capacity to reflect on the child's internal experience is a key indicator of the parent's reflective capacity to be mind-minded (Meins, 1998). Similar concepts like 'reflective functioning' describe the parent's capacity to mentalise others' mental states, intentions, feelings, thoughts and beliefs.

CASE STUDY F

Child F was 3 years old when the assessment took place in the kinship carer's home, where he had been living for 6 weeks since the death of his mother. The kinship carer was a relative of F's father, who lived abroad, and had not known F's mother well.

The kinship carer was sensitive to F's distress and described how F had called and cried out for his mother initially for the first month. The carer moved between being very attuned to F's emotional state and how it was affecting his eating and capacity to accept comfort, to being more distant and a little dismissive saying F was now 'fine'.

After we observed F become very fearful of a doll that was 'sleeping' we explored the meaning of this for F. We could see that it was upsetting him despite the fact he was so quiet at these moments (the family had been treating it as a 'joke', not realising the significance). The carer recalled that a relative had told F that his mother was now 'sleeping'. A discussion led to a more sensitive response from the carer, and she went on to help support F when anxious, developing a gentle approach that allowed F to have a different relationship with this symbolic object. Over the next weeks, F became able to play ordinary domestic games that included the doll, and his eating habits improved alongside. ●●●

The structured DASS questionnaire focuses on questions that relate to the parent's current levels of stress, anxiety and depression. It can be a starting point when a parent wishes to share more about wider experiences and how these impact on their well-being, health, relationships and daily life.

In addition, when discussing the final question on the ASQ:SE with the parent, which asks about what they enjoy most about their child, we can hear differences in the quality of the response. These can be detailed or very general descriptions. Sometimes answers reveal a distorted perspective, for example, when the parent moves quickly to mentioning only negative themes or characteristics that are inappropriate to the child's age, or may not be observable to the worker.

Child's individual development

EXPLORING A CHILD'S HISTORY

Taking a history about the child's early health and development, from prenatal to the present, helps to inform our understanding of influences and experiences from their past, e.g. prenatal conditions for baby or mother, stressors in pregnancy, birth history, post-natal progress, etc. Using a standard template helps this to be as thorough and focused as possible and it is transparent to the parent that these are routine questions. Exploring this history will inevitably raise the inextricably linked experiences of the mother, and father, at these key developmental times. There is wide variation in how parents recount the history of their child's early development, with issues ranging from memories being raised of a previously difficult time to the parent's current mental and emotional state affecting the capacity to recall and provide any detailed information. There can be information that only comes to light later as the work progresses and memories are evoked and shared.

If the parent has given clear permission for the team to have access to additional reports and information from the network, this can be used to build the background picture of the child. This information may reveal other important influences on the child pre- or post-natally such as exposure to drugs or alcohol in pregnancy, or domestic abuse. Domestic abuse is now described as one of the forms of child abuse and can have a direct and indirect impact on the child's safety and well-being similar to other forms of abuse (Myers et al., 2002). Consideration needs to be given to how and when any new information is acknowledged with a parent that has not been directly reported by them, but learned through access to other reports.

A standardised questionnaire on the child's social-emotional development is one of the measures that looks in detail at the individual child's progress and difficulties. The ASQ:SE is accessible to parents and is useful in providing rich data when delivered as a semi-structured interview (Hardy et al., 2015). Through discussion about their responses to specific questions, the parent is encouraged to give everyday examples of the child's mastery of, or difficulties with, the developmental tasks applicable to their age. This can provide insight into the responses the parent makes about behaviours, and the strategies that the parent employs to cope with or support their child. For example, a child who cannot settle at night is also described as disliking being held or cuddled and does not make any reference to their parent in a new environment, which demonstrates conflict in the child's attachment and being emotionally reliant on others. The discussions can also give insight into the child's presentation when expected behaviours for the child's age are absent or infrequent, resulting in a score of '0' on the measure. For example, a child does not score any points for the 'prolonged crying' item, but on discussion the caregiver describes that the child never cries at all, even when hurt or hungry.

DISCUSSION AND CLARIFICATION

As there is common ground across some of the questions, it is possible to see where there may be confirmation of behaviour in a later answer. Conversely, there may be inconsistencies or contradictions from one answer to another. This can then lead to further exploration with the parent, e.g. a foster parent who initially describes the child as signalling their needs but later reports that they are predicting what the child wants as the child does not actually communicate their needs. As structured questionnaires require a concrete response to an individual item, there is the possibility that an answer may suggest that there is no concern in relation to a defined behaviour. For example, the parent describes that the child likes to be hugged/cuddled but also reports that the child never initiates physical contact and cries inconsolably. The discussion may then elaborate this issue further and hear of concerns that will not be highlighted by the questionnaire responses alone. Similarly if a child's responses are frequently absent in one area, this can be explored in more depth around other questions that may reveal this occurring in different areas of functioning. For example, an infant who rarely cries or protests, and who does not have overt sleeping difficulties, but on further exploration is described as being unusually quiet for long periods in their cot on waking.

Direct observation of the child will help inform the therapist in relation to specific questions and explanations of when and why behaviours occur, which may contrast with the parent's view. For example, a child who immediately walks away from their parent in a new situation but who was reported in response to the questionnaire item as always checking their parent's presence, may lead to a discussion and the parent adjusting their rating of the item and their understanding.

Throughout the delivery of parent-report questionnaires, we can reflect with the parent about the history of a particular behaviour or response. This can highlight positive changes which is encouraging when a parent may be feeling overwhelmed and anxious overall. It can reveal how serious the infant/child's earlier responses were, e.g. a baby who did not register pain, or another who slept for the vast majority of day and night. It also provides awareness of what areas of functioning may hold particular vulnerability for the child in future should they experience heightened stress or further trauma/neglect.

DEVELOPMENTAL SCREENING

The use of a developmental screening, such as the Denver II, provides important feedback on general aspects of the child's functioning in the following domains:

- personal–social
- fine motor
- gross motor
- language.

It is a part of the assessment that parents are often keen to engage with as most parents want their child to progress well and are looking for confirmation and reassurance about this. Where specific strengths are highlighted, this is encouraging and a source of pride and pleasure for the parents. Equally if the child is having difficulties in one or more specific domains, consideration of how it relates to the developmental profile as a whole can be given, and will be integrated into the final feedback and be delivered in a clear but thoughtful way.

By providing information on the specific areas of the child's general development, the Denver II has parallel uses.

- Firstly, it is an opportunity for the therapist to have some direct interaction with the child, though this is done in conjunction with the parent's involvement in a way that does not undermine the parent's central role. We would check the parent's view on what approach would facilitate the engagement of the child. This can reveal where the parent places the importance of their own involvement, and what role they feel they have in facilitating their child's activity and participation. Some parents can adapt flexibly and support the child, organising the environment to help facilitate the process. For others, they may either withdraw (offering little or no attention or reassurance) or become intrusive (giving the child the answers or making pressurising or negative comments).
- In addition it provides insight into how the child manages to focus, co-operate and accept support to complete the tasks including those which are challenging.

The profile of the child's abilities from the Denver II shows whether there are specific aspects of development that are of concern alongside the social-emotional and relationship presentations. In many cases there is a varied picture, but it may reveal that the child's general functioning is on track with specific delays and problems mostly in their social-emotional functioning and attachment. Sometimes there are clear links between specific presenting relationship patterns and an identified developmental concern. For example, a child and parent who are finding it hard to emotionally separate may be exacerbating gross motor delays, or a parent who rarely communicates with their child can be linked to a delay on the language sub-scale.

CASE STUDY G

Child G was a 2 and a half year-old girl who lived with her father and her mother, who had longstanding physical and mental health difficulties. She excelled in each area of the Denver, particularly in the language domain where she was able to complete tasks well above her expected age. Her mum was very proud of her daughter's abilities and spoke of 'forgetting' that she was not yet 3 years old and how she could treat her like an older child.

Difficulties were described by her parents through the ASQ:SE where many concerns about G's behaviour and emotional responses emerged. These included frequent long tantrums, biting, throwing toys, running away from her mum when out, and 'anxiety attacks' where she would become very difficult to comfort. ●●●

Clinical observations of the child occur through the visits and include the child's:

- predominant emotional expression/state
- pattern of mood changes
- presence of emotional regulation
- responses to parental involvement or withdrawal.

The child's emotional and social response to the therapist is important and although care is taken not to take over or undermine the parent we may see the effects of brief interactions in terms of the child's responsiveness, regulation or triggering of anxiety.

Some symptomatic presentations can be noted which may not have been reported directly by parents, for example:

- signs of dissociation
- freezing
- sexualised behaviour
- harm to self or others
- animal cruelty
- compulsive tidying and cleaning.

Figure 4.6 on the next page is a visual representation of the confusing clinical presentations, that although initially may appear random, can be

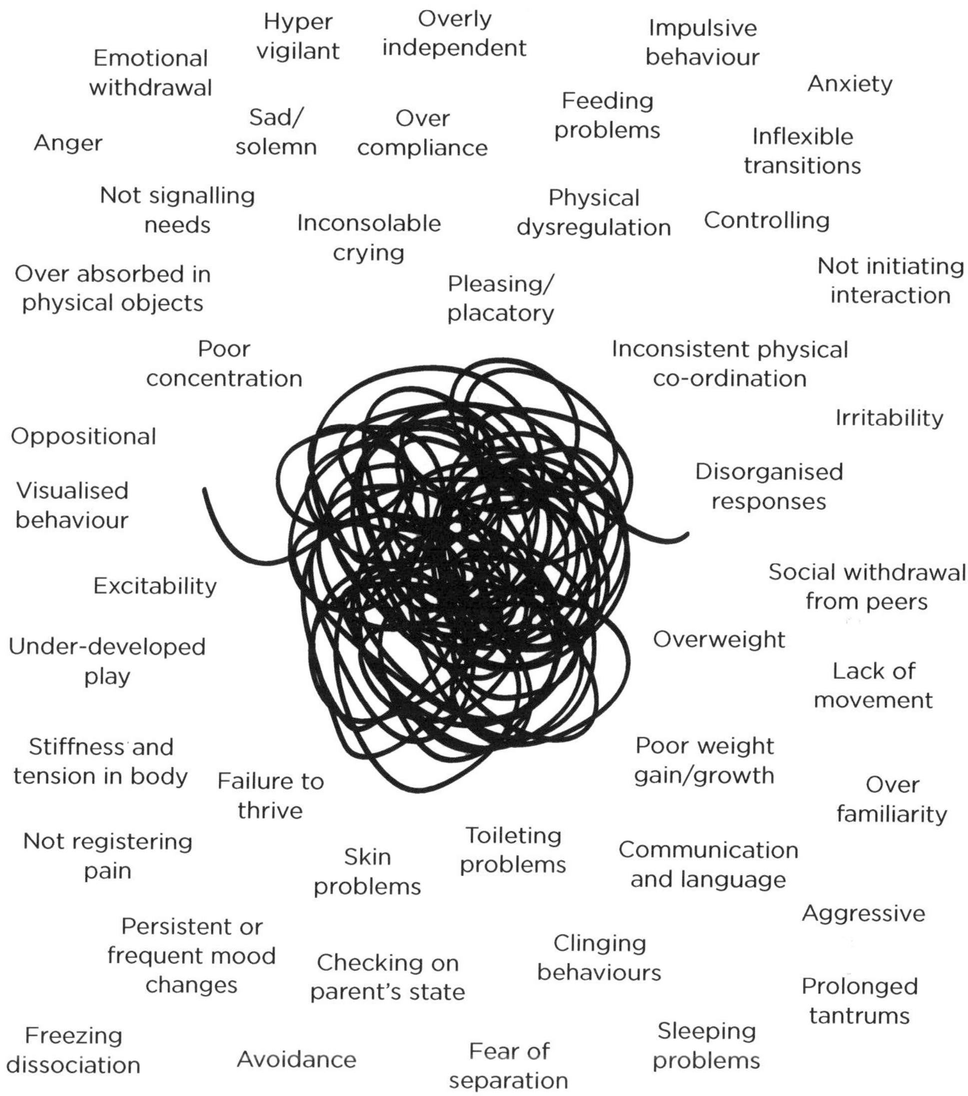

Figure 4.6 Clinical features observed in assessments

understood if the therapist is prepared to accept contradictory features that represent the child's inner state.

A therapist's capacity to enter into the emotional experience of the child is a vital ingredient in interpreting the child's state and containing and verbalising this in such a way that the parent might be able to think about it (Bion, 1962b).

Emotional	Behavioural	Functional	Physical	Child-parent interaction
Emotional withdrawal	Prolonged tantrums	Sleeping problems	Skin problems	Checking on parent's state
Anxiety	Inconsolable crying	Under-developed play	Failure to thrive	Pleasing/placatory
Solemn/sad	Persistent or frequent mood changes	Inflexible transitions	Overweight	Disorganised responses
Persistent or frequent mood changes	Overly independent	Inconsistent physical co-ordination	Poor weight gain/growth	Over compliance
Emotional withdrawal	Irritability	Poor concentration, communication and language	Not registering pain	Avoidance
Hyper-vigilant	Controlling	Feeding problems	Lack of movement	Not signalling needs
	Physical dysregulation	Toileting problems	Stiffness and tension in the body	Clinging behaviours
	Oppositional	Not initiating interaction		Fear of separation
	Impulsive behaviour	Social withdrawal from peers		Over-absorbed by physical objects
	Blank or flat expression			
	Aggressive			
	Sexualised behaviour			
	Excitability			

Figure 4.7 Clinical features, categorised

Figure 4.7 illustrates how the observed clinical features can be clustered in key domains to give a profile of the child's own clinical presentation and the relationship with their parent. It helps to more clearly define and separate out problem areas which can later be used to inform the intervention.

Emotional	Behavioural	Functional	Physical	Child-parent interaction
Child 1: 3 m Emotional withdrawal	Inconsolable crying Blank or flat expression	Sleeping problems Not initiating interaction Feeding problems	Stiffness and tension in body	Avoidance Not signalling needs
Child 2: 9 m Anxiety Solemn/sad	Blank or flat expression	Feeding problems Under-developed play Not initiating interaction	Stiffness and tension in body Skin problems Overweight Not registering pain Lack of movement	Over compliance Disorganised responses Not signalling needs
Child 3: 9 m Anger	Controlling Physical dysregulation Aggression to self Blank or flat expression	Feeding problems	Asthma/other conditions Stiffness and tension in body	Avoidance
Child 4: 3y 4 m Persistent or frequent mood changes	Prolonged tantrums Oppositional Aggressive Excitability	Poor concentration Difficulties with peers Feeding problems	Asthma/other conditions	Intrusive/ demanding Clinging behaviours

Figure 4.8 Composite examples of children's clinical features at assessment.

In Figure 4.8 a visual mapping of composite case profiles shows the variety and range of needs in babies and young children at assessment. In clinical practice, this mapping can be repeated as treatment progresses to note changes. Work continues on this clinical profiling and will be reported on in future papers.

Formulation and report writing

The information from the assessment visits and any additional information gained from the wider network were collated by the CAMHS therapist to produce a written summary report. This highlighted strengths and difficulties in the child's social-emotional development, relationships, mental health and general developmental needs, along with a formulation and recommendations.

Reports were designed to be brief and factual, using ordinary language in order to be accessible. They combined specific feedback from the measures as well as a narrative that incorporated the parent and child's experience as we observed and heard this. A report template was developed and used to structure the format and core components that needed to be covered. It can be found on page 93.

Feedback meeting to family and network

On completion of the assessment report, the therapist arranged a feedback meeting with the parent(s) or carer who completed the assessment and with key workers in the child and family's network.

In circumstances where the child was no longer living with the birth parent, a separate meeting was arranged to discuss the child's presentation and needs, with a particular focus on suggestions and advice for the contact time between the birth parent and child. The feedback meeting included the birth parent where possible, always involved the child's social worker and often included the designated contact worker. If it was not possible to meet with the contact worker in person, relevant information could be shared, and further liaison to talk through how they could facilitate the recommendations with parent and child.

The style of the report was important as it required factual details of the child's emotional and general development, as well as references to the relationship; noting the contribution by the child and patterns of interaction that might be affecting the child on an emotional and functional level. It also needed to acknowledge the impact of the pressures and adversity on the parent(s) and be sensitive to their experience of guilt, anxiety or denial about the issues and concerns highlighted.

During the feedback meeting, discussion focused on the family's response to the content of the report, including the recommendations, with time to think further about any intervention being offered. This gave an opportunity to:

- describe practical aspects of the intervention, e.g. typically consisting of weekly hour-long sessions at their preferred location
- talk about the duration of the intervention, i.e. up to 15 sessions for birth parents and 10 for foster carers were delivered in the projects.

Some of the caregivers we worked with in our clinical service were new early permanence carers, kinship carers or prospective adopters and they would typically be offered the longer intervention as they were likely to be in a long-term parental role to the child.

Some families were offered a reduced intervention of approximately six sessions as appropriate to the level of need identified. Parents' responses to the assessment reports were found to be highly individual and varied in terms of how much they agreed with the formulation. The great majority thought that we had described their child and the relationship in a balanced and accurate way. However, as the reports often referenced some difficult or painful issues, the feedback needed to be delivered in a thoughtful and sensitive way. The meeting provided a space to consider new ways of thinking about the child and their relationship and to consider whether they wished to continue to work with us where an intervention was recommended. Some parents needed time to consider their decision and further discussion.

For some families the assessment and feedback sessions were considered to be an intervention in themselves. They created sufficient shifts in the parent's understanding of their relationship with their child and the child's needs, to support them to make changes and feel greater confidence in going forwards with these.

The feedback meeting also gave professionals new information about the child's emotional well-being and mental health that had relevance to care planning or community support packages. Discussions with the professionals and family considered how the information on the child's specific needs could be translated into advice for other people in the network or new carers. This often led to the therapist developing an individual Activity template about specific approaches that others could use to engage with the child and support their social-emotional development further, e.g. for birth parents in contact sessions or teachers/nursery workers in schools. (An example of an Assessment report template is shown on the next page and an editable version can be downloaded from www.susiweb.co.uk.)

Conclusion

We have all heard the expression 'they will grow out of it'. Indeed most of us would avoid intervening unnecessarily and disrupting the parent and child's developing bond which is tested in most ordinary circumstances by fatigue, worry and responsibility brought by parenthood. However, this can inhibit an exploration and identification of problems that do exist, due to concern that we might cause the parent more stress and a sense of being blamed. A further factor is that it is complicated to reach a formulation about young children's progress when there are early but subtle signs of difficulty, not recognised by the parent themselves, or which could easily be seen as 'a passing phase'.

In this early developmental phase we see clear indicators for later emotional, behavioural and developmental difficulties but lack evidenced assessment procedures to use in clinical practice (Moriarty, Baginsky, Gorin, Baginsky & Manthorpe, 2016). Clinical evidence from the SUSI study goes some way to addressing this gap.

Name of service: ____________________

Address: ____________________

SUSI Assessment template

Name: ____________________ **DOB:** __________

Date of assessment: __________ **Age of child at assessment:** __________

Location of screening: ____________________

Informants: ____________________ **Relationship to child:** __________

General information

The children and parents complete a range of standardised and reliable measures, including the Ages & Stages Questionnaire: Social-emotional (ASQ:SE), as part of this assessment. These measures contribute to the profile of the child's developmental and social-emotional needs.

In thinking about the results from the questionnaires, and home visit where applicable, we have considered other factors and information available to us including the child's health and general development, the timing of the screening, and cultural factors.

Any specific comments or concerns that have been shared with us by parents or carers during the assessment have also contributed to this profile of the child and any recommendations we may make.

Assessment feedback:

____

____

Summary and recommendations:

____

____

Signed by: [therapist's signature]

____

____

5 Intervention

The intervention has helped us understand our son better and think about his behaviour without pathologising him. It supported us both directly in the sessions and gave guidance for us at home. The therapist listened to us and it's helped us put our son's needs in context.

PARENT

The aim of the intervention is to promote the social-emotional development of the infant or young child, and their relationships and attachment to their main caregiver(s). The parent-child approach used is based on the principle that the caregiver-child relationship is the main agent for change. The work to support and develop this relationship best meets the specific needs of the infant/child now, as well as building social-emotional security and wider developmental benefits for the future. The intervention is informed by clinical research and practice, and draws on infant/child development, attachment, systemic and psychoanalytic theories.

Each intervention is tailored to the individual child and their relationship to their primary caregiver(s), with the adult's experience of the child and relationship being supported and explored. It is informed by the assessment, and the structure and delivery includes a combination of:

- **parent-child relationship 'live' work:**
  - using spontaneous interactions in play-based sessions (structured and/or non-directive)
  - focusing on specific communications and interactions that are adaptive and promote the parent-child relationship
  - promoting parental thoughtfulness through exploration of the child's specific responses and behaviours that signal the child's underlying mental and emotional states
  - addressing maladaptive patterns of interaction

- **reflective discussion with parents to:**
  - discuss current experiences of parenting and their relationship with their child
  - explore the links between past and present experiences linked to the relationship and the child's needs
- **liaison and joint work with other networks to:**
  - share an understanding of the child's needs with the wider family and/or network
  - develop multi-agency care plans as needed.

Similar to the assessment process, the intervention was delivered in a variety of community bases. Most often this was in the family home (the preferred location for the family would have been discussed and planned in the feedback session). Some families who completed the assessment in their homes chose to go to a local Children's Centre or come to the clinic base for the intervention for a variety of reasons. (This flexibility was, and continues to be, an important factor in retaining the families' engagement.) There are advantages to delivering an intervention in either the family home or in other more neutral settings, and some adaptation to the therapeutic techniques and the practical application of these are needed in each.

The stages of the intervention process are described below. Specific techniques used within the three different phases (initial, central and ending) are referred to. The therapeutic techniques will be described in detail within each phase, along with case examples to illustrate how they are used in practice.

Initial sessions: engagement and establishing the focus

The process of engagement with the parent(s) will have begun when first meeting them to discuss joining the project or clinical service. It continues throughout the intervention stage, and follow-up reviews. It is likely, and preferable in most cases, that the therapist delivering the intervention will have undertaken the assessment. In this way they will have established some rapport and trust with the family, having demonstrated empathy and a capacity to contain the parent's and child's feelings and states during the earlier assessment visits. When this is not possible or appropriate, the therapist joining to work with the family for the intervention should try to attend the feedback session along with the colleague who carried out the assessment. Time can then be given to talking about the experience of the assessment and the parent's priorities in starting the intervention, being mindful of the child's needs highlighted by the assessment.

When working with parents and very young children, the therapist needs to keep a balanced and even-handed approach in attending to both the parent's emotional states as well as reflecting on the child's possible feelings; the timing for the articulation of these for each individual requires consideration according to the level of mind-mindedness that the parent demonstrates.

Following the feedback meeting, it is important during the first session or two to establish an initial focus with the parent on one or more issues identified in the assessment. There is also a need to manage the expectations, anxieties and conflicts that can arise around the start of therapy. The role of the therapist is to provide emotional support and understanding to the parent and child, and to start to facilitate change at this stage. For some parents the opportunity to start this process of change is a positive and hopeful experience, but for others it can raise anxieties about their role and capacity to change. It is important to think together about the timescale of the work at this point: while it will have been discussed previously in the feedback meeting, it will underline for the parent that this is a time-limited piece of work. (For many families this can help them to engage as it is experienced as less overwhelming than a longer-term commitment.)

In the initial sessions it is important to be open to hearing about any immediate issues that have arisen since the feedback meeting. These may communicate new information about the family, or sometimes a conflict has arisen more clearly about the lens being on the child or relationship. Parents may express feeling hopeless or frustrated about other external preoccupations or want to talk about their own thoughts/feelings and feel conflicted about sharing the space and time with their child. Sensitivity to this is needed while also keeping the primary focus on the relationship.

It is helpful to discuss and negotiate with the parent:

- how many sessions are available
- the general aims for the intervention
- an agreed focus for the first sessions.

This demonstrates that the intervention has a flexible structure. (It was found that parents felt contained by knowing that there were boundaries and an end-point, especially those who had not previously experienced therapeutic work, recognising too that the end of the work raises its own issues.)

The two main starting points for the intervention are either beginning with direct live parent–child work, or to have some reflective discussion and/or psychoeducation with the parent. This decision will be reached in response to the views that the parent expresses in the feedback and subsequent conversation about the intervention offer. For example:

- some parents feel that they have shared a lot of their history in the assessment and wish to turn to the direct work with their child, while being aware that individual time will be available to them to explore issues further at a later stage in the intervention
- other parents benefit from some space to explore their own experience and thoughts about what encompasses emotional development and child attachment as these may be 'new' concepts to them.

Engagement techniques

CREATING A COMFORTABLE ENVIRONMENT

It is important to create a 'space' that is as comfortable as possible for the parent and the child to occupy. This will have been considered in the discussion about where and when to carry out the intervention. Many dyads benefit from a quiet, contained room, particularly if the baby or child is easily distracted or avoidant. While this is not always possible in the first instance, it can form part of the discussions with the parent, and sometimes leads to the parent choosing another environment or time for the work, e.g. moving the sessions from the home to a room in the Children's Centre or nursery.

THERAPIST AS FACILITATOR (NOT PARTICIPANT)

The role of the therapist towards the parent and child will be discussed in the feedback meeting and early sessions. The aim is to highlight the importance of the therapist's role as a facilitator rather than as an active participant in the relationship or with the child. Some parents and children may be operating in a distant or disconnected way, so the therapist needs to devise ways to make them feel most at ease. At the same time, they need to create opportunities for them to interact in a way that helps them to make progress in small steps. For example, a parent may suggest that the child sits with the therapist, or places the buggy at the far end of the room, or places a table between themselves and their child: this requires the therapist to suggest that the parent and child be within reach or sight of one another while at the same time gauging the proximity and intensity that they are able to manage at this point. Little may be said overtly as these are early days and a supportive approach can often be appropriate with limited exploration at this stage. General statements about the therapist not actively initiating interaction with the baby/child are often helpful, as the parent–child relationship is the one to be supported. (Or an explanation can be offered as to why the therapist is not joining with the child's play or chat.) The therapist will gently tell the child to approach or turn to the parent rather than them to establish this foundation.

SHARING FOCUS AND IDEAS

The aim is to create a space where the parent and therapist can have a shared focus on the child, and jointly share ideas. A reflective space may be a relatively new experience, so the pace of the work needs to be flexible. The therapist and parent may reflect on the issues relating to where the focus/work might begin, and reiterate the general non-directive approach. With this acknowledgement that the more open 'free' quality of intervention sessions may feel different to other experiences they have had, there is the chance to talk through doubts and worries along the way together. As the sessions progress, the emphasis is on the parent and therapist getting to know what can work for the family. Some reassurance/containment may be needed if the parent feels compelled to be very active or demanding of the child and behave in certain defensive ways. This helps to create a child-centred focus and establishes the importance of the parent's view and role.

EMOTIONAL CONTAINMENT

The child's and parent's strategies to cope emotionally in the session may be similar to those shown in the assessment, but they might also reveal new anxieties or defences (coping mechanisms). The parent may feel pressure to make the child manage differently to usual. In the less structured time of the intervention session you may see how frequently the child and parent need 'time out' from interacting with one another to down-regulate. New insights from these initial sessions can help to inform the work and become explicitly part of the shared agenda early on, or can be revisited when the therapeutic relationship is more established.

Central intervention sessions

The main body of the intervention focuses on the quality of the parent-child relationship and how through supported and facilitated change, this relationship can then best meet the current emotional and developmental needs of the child.

This period of the work involves the ongoing evolution of reciprocal emotional and behavioural cycles between the parent and child. This builds a strong foundation for future stages of development and relationships. The dyadic relationship is explored through both direct work on the 'live' parent-child interaction as well as reflective discussion and developmental guidance with the parent. In addition, specific recommendations for the approach to and care of the child may be made to key workers in the network, in collaboration with other family members or professionals. This would usually take place towards the end of this stage of work, when some changes have occurred, and when the parent feels clearer and more comfortable about what they might wish to share with others. Exceptions to this may be in circumstances where there is a legal or safeguarding context in which interim feedback is required.

While the parent has a greater role and responsibility for bringing about change to improve the quality of the relationship with their child, this approach recognises the child as an active contributor to the blocks in interaction and the opportunities for change. The detailed assessment gives an insight and working hypothesis about how the child's coping mechanisms are adaptive to the immediate context of the relationship; it also points to ways in which the cycle of relating to others has become unhelpful to their progress and development now, and possibly in the future.

As well as the focus on the micro-interactions between parent and child and reflective discussions with the parent, other resources may be integrated into the work such as:

- the model's specific written/visual handouts
- video clips of infant development
- 'homework' ideas
- viewing the family's own videos.

These will be covered in later sections of this chapter and in Chapter 6, with examples of when they may be useful to introduce to parents and integrate into the work.

A therapist's presence with a parent/child dyad introduces a third person into the dynamic. This can bring triangulation issues to the fore that are commonly found in work with couples or siblings. In our work there are two individuals who have, externally at least, very different levels of responsibility, maturity and control. On the other hand they may be experiencing intense feelings of vulnerability in their own right, as well as rivalry for the therapist's attention. When strong, primitive emotions are stirred up in both parent and child, interactions between them can be intensely emotional and unpredictable. The containing space of the therapy can be structured when necessary to provide boundaries and to pace the intensity of the work. This moves between supporting the relationship to develop in the 'here and now' and exploring the representations that the child and parent have of each other. As the babies and children are so young, this occurs to different degrees across the age spans from 0–4 years and will be illustrated with case examples below.

Eleven broad themes were identified that therapists would cover during the course of the intervention (see Figure 5.1 on the next page), with corresponding written and visual resources.

The themes are described in detail in Chapter 6. The resources relating to the themes are described later in this chapter (see 'Techniques with parents') and they are available via an online system (see page 16 of the Introduction for a link to these resources).

The themes for sessions provided a framework for:

- promoting parent–child interaction
- increasing a parent's capacity to recognise and be attuned to their child's emotional/mental states
- exploring 'blocks' in communicating with and relating to one another for both parent and child.

The themes are tailored to each family but are not delivered in a linear structured way; they are used with the therapeutic techniques to explore and support the child–parent relationship.

The practical approaches to help the parent/child dyad effect change are tailored initially to the assessment findings and then reviewed according to:

- the family's response to treatment
- the parent's mental states
- other contextual factors.

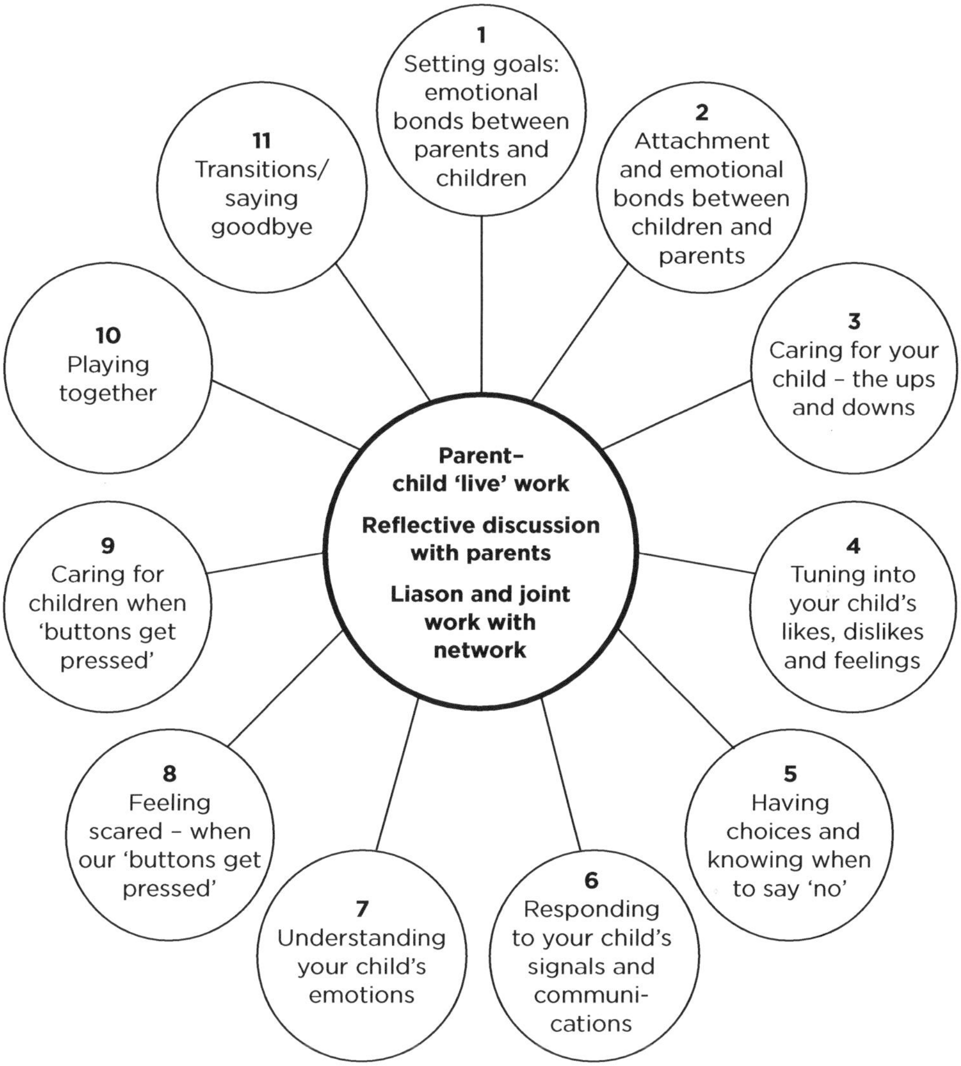

Figure 5.1 Intervention themes

In the sections that follow, the three core approaches are described:

1. **parent–child relationship 'live' work**, along with techniques that can be used to support change in the parent–child relationship
2. **reflective work with the parent** – in practice this often co-occurs with the live work (as illustrated by some of the clinical scenarios)
3. **liaison with the network** – this is described more fully in Chapter 8 although examples are given within the sections below of the practical ways that information about the child's and parent's needs were shared to inform other family members and professionals about the approach to the child and attachment relationship(s).

At the end of the chapter there are descriptions of how the work is tailored in different contexts and to specific populations.

1 Parent–child relationship 'live' work

Considerable challenges are experienced by babies and young children who have a history of not having an adult who can help them to:

- regulate themselves emotionally and physically adequately
- develop the trust and security that their needs and feelings will be thought about and responded to.

Babies develop adaptive responses in which they attempt to match the mindset of their primary caregiver. This results in them trying to manage their own emotional and physical states in a range of ways. For example, they will 'up-regulate' (crying, fussing, clinging) or 'down-regulate' (avoidant, blank, undemanding) in an unconscious effort to match the mental coping strategy of the parent.

When parents struggle with their own stressors, and fluctuating, poorly-regulated mental/emotional states in parallel with their child, they can be overwhelmed (to differing degrees) by the feelings or sense of vulnerability that their baby expresses and evokes in them. If the parent has no experience of being helped to regulate and understand their feelings, and/or is currently living with chronic stress, they are operating at either a high state of arousal or conversely a dampened down state. In these contexts, the parent's capacity to think about and manage their own and their young child's feelings can be affected and at times severely compromised.

Another common situation is one where the parent has been affected by a period of ill health or stress, and has recovered, but the baby/child continues to show the same responses (internalised from the earlier stage of relationship with parent). These responses have now become maladaptive, e.g. lack of responsivity to the now more available parent. This can create stress and distress for the parent, in turn creating further negative cycles whereby parents become depressed by the awareness of how their relationship with their baby has been impacted. Similar patterns can be seen for young children moving from one primary caregiver to another, e.g. birth parent to foster carer: the child activates a system of relating with the new caregiver that mirrors the familiar cycles of relating that they had with their parent (Stovall-McClough & Dozier, 2004).

TECHNIQUES FOR PARENT–CHILD 'LIVE' WORK

1. Observations about micro-interactions

In this technique, the therapist gives the parent a commentary about their observations of the child, of the parent's involvement and efforts, as well as the child's response. The brief narratives have many purposes and need to be oriented to the type/levels of interactions and closeness that the child and parent managed in the assessment.

Firstly, the therapist gives the parent the message that they are interested and attending to them and their relationship. The therapist also engages the parent to be alongside them in their thoughts about the child as well as themselves as a parent.

CASE STUDY H

Child H, aged 3 and a half years, demanded her mother's attention constantly in the early sessions, becoming highly active and anxious if any reference was made to the child. As her mother was also in a high state of emotional arousal, short comments were made in sessions to steer her focus back to her daughter regularly. Separate parallel discussions with mother were needed from the outset to help her reflect on H's needs and her responses and feelings to H. ●●●

The commentary also has the goal of establishing a shared language so that the therapist uses words that fit with the parent's usual way of describing states and emotions. It also introduces ways of putting into words experiences and feelings that the parent may not ordinarily articulate. This approach can begin to highlight the times when a child's changing behaviour may indicate an underlying feeling state, or a shift in their regulatory state, seen in changes of physical and/or emotional responses. Some of these individual or interactional behaviours may be new or unusual for the child and naming them can help to bring them to the attention and awareness of the parent.

CASE STUDY I

Child I, aged 5 months, presented with frequent behaviours indicative of underlying tensions, such as arching his back and pushing away from his parent. The parent attributed these to the baby wanting to stand up by himself. Comments to the parent to acknowledge this belief, together with alternative ideas about the baby's state and need to down-regulate (helping to bring awareness of the mind–body link), began to influence the parent's approach to him. This was important as the baby appeared to have a number of somatic responses to stress with episodes of eczema occurring at times of heightened tension between parent and child. ●●●

There are obvious benefits of highlighting positive responses that a child may make towards the parent, and the parent may be ready to hear this and be pleased. In turn, this elicits a positive cycle of interaction with their response. However, if a parent responds by rejecting the therapist's observation, think about the pace at which the parent can receive information that challenges their current attributions to the child and themselves; it indicates that further sensitive exploration is needed. The example below also illustrates the complexity of mixed feelings for a parent who experiences something positive but new with their child.

CASE STUDY J

Child J was 14 months old. In an early intervention session, she moved to sit with her mother soon after mum had reflected aloud on how difficult J found one to one interaction. She did not appear to notice that she had become so close until this was commented on by the therapist. Mum looked emotional and said that this was the first time J had initiated this. The intervention built on the new ways of relating by supporting the interactions moment to moment. ●●●

2. Supporting new interactions and communication between parent and child

When the parent and therapist have established a way of talking about the micro-interactions between the parent and child, ideas can be introduced as a natural situation arises. This can include suggesting small changes, or things to add into their involvement together, both practically and emotionally.

There are inherent risks within this process that one of the dyad will reject the offer of interest or closer contact from the other. However, with the therapist's containment, these are also opportunities to relate differently and safely with another person (the therapist) to support them. The therapist may begin by making an observation, e.g. a cue from the child that they are motivated to share something with the parent but are unsure whether to approach them. The positive intent may be remarked on, rather than the ambivalence and, by prompting the parent to notice, there is the chance for a new cycle of interaction to take place. Often this requires a 'light touch' so that pressure or emotional intensity is not added to a situation that may already be anxiety-provoking for both the child and parent.

There are many different ways and contexts in which this technique can be introduced. In itself it is a process that develops between the therapist and the dyad, with particular sensitivity to the parent's and child's states at the time. There may have been specific conversations already that have unpicked some of the meaning in a behaviour that the parent has expressed concern about, or that the therapist has noted as being distressing/ difficult for parent and child. The therapist may need to flag up when a particular interaction is repeated and check that the parent could be open to thinking about it further. The timing is important so that the parent is gently challenged to focus on the child and their own responses but feels supported by the therapist to do so. This is because, at times, this may conflict with their wish to talk about their own preoccupations and issues.

The approaches in Figures 5.2 and 5.3 on the next page are divided between communications from the therapist to the child, and to the parent. They may be used alongside one another because both parties need support from the therapist to engage in unfamiliar ways of relating. Parent and child alike are exploring how these different interactions are possible and can feel 'safe'.

Some parents may only be able to engage in limited discussion about their underlying feelings and needs or those of their child. However, they are motivated to support their child, and starting the intervention is evidence that they are open, in some ways, to new ideas. In these contexts, the therapist will suggest small ways that the parent could interact in the moment, e.g. introducing some phrases to respond to their baby's babble.

CASE STUDY K

Child K, aged 2 and a half years, showed subtle signs of ongoing distress when she accidentally broke a toy; the foster parent did not initially register how upset the child was. The therapist prompted the carer to continue to offer support and verbal reassurance for a longer period than we'd observed they would normally do. Sensitive feedback was given to the carer about how the child responded to this positively, noting with them the behavioural signs that the child needed an extended period of support to fully calm and settle. This helped the foster parent to continue to offer support in this way when needed by the child. ●●●

The therapist may comment on how they notice the child is feeling, focusing on as many positive responses as possible but also making gentle reference to the child feeling distressed, 'she looked a bit upset there'. This feedback can be built on to make links between the feeling state and the interactional context, 'she looked a bit upset when the game was over and you had to sort out her bottle'.

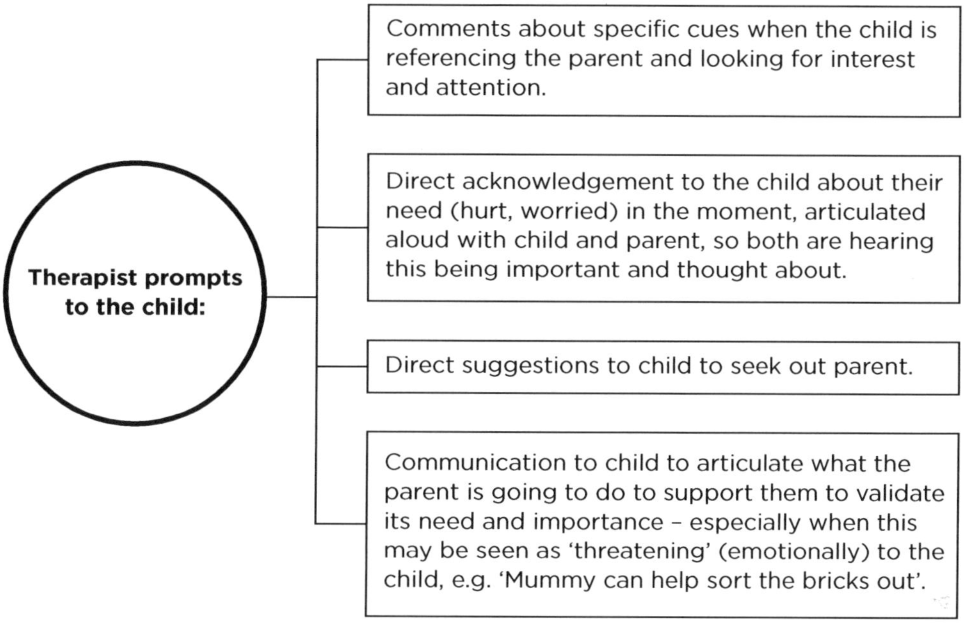

Figure 5.2 Communication from the therapist to the child

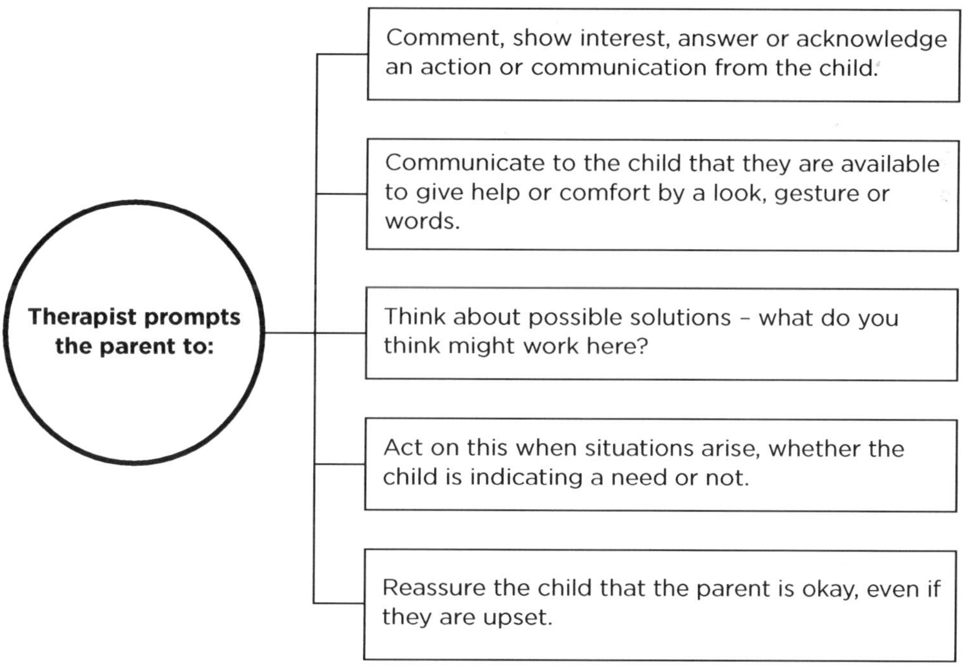

Figure 5.3 Communication from the therapist to the parent

CASE STUDY L

Child L, aged 6 months, was observed to be remote with her new kinship carer and communicated few signs of need. The therapist's comments focused on small responses that the child made that indicated her connection with her carer, e.g. smiling as her carer approached her, fleeting frowns at other moments. The carer was encouraged to make a gentle commentary to the child about her actions, wishes and feelings more generally. This needed prompts and support from the therapist until it was more established and the baby started to give more spontaneous feedback to her carer. ●●●

The next step may be to help the parent think how they can be available in different ways through transition and times of change of focus, however small. The child who is beginning to invest more in the relationship may be particularly sensitive to the parent withdrawing, even momentarily. At this stage of the process, consider how the child's heightened demands may be impacting on the parent. It is usually helpful to identify and discuss the greater demand on them emotionally, which can bring rewards but also challenges, triggering underlying anxiety or feelings of vulnerability and rivalry. It may be that the child's new behaviours and communications are attributed with a negative connotation, e.g. more clingy or aggressive, and this will then need to be explored and worked with.

CASE STUDY M

Child M, 11 months, was very avoidant of her parent in general, with outbursts of intense distress at bedtimes. The therapist and mother thought about how to pick up on small cues in the daytime that indicated the child needed a response or some soothing. As interactions quickly became very excitable, the therapist helped mum to regulate her own emotional state and supported her to try quieter, calming responses to her baby. This led to the mother being more engaged in general with M, and reflections on how this affected her emotionally and practically. ●●●

THERAPIST'S INTERACTION WITH CHILD

The primary goal of the intervention is to promote and support the relationship between the child and the parent, so careful thought is needed as to how the therapist positions themselves in relation to the child. The therapist will have stated that the relationship between the parent and the child is the pivotal one. They will have stressed that they are there as a facilitator, and that building a relationship with the child is not a significant aspect of the work.

However, the therapist needs to find a way in which they can relate to the child that assists the main goal of supporting the child–parent relationship. They need to use their observations of, and communications from, the child to raise awareness and insight into how the child experiences the relationship with their parent. There will be times when an informed decision is made to introduce more direct communications or activity with the child (usually with children from 3 years or older). However, this approach would always take place with the planned and active involvement of the parent in the session and would only be for a time limited period.

CASE STUDY N

Child N was 3 years old. He had recently experienced the death of his mother. During the intervention, the therapist engaged in direct work using symbolic play with N. As the issues of loss were also painful for his kinship carer, the therapist took the lead but supported the carer to join in with the play and discussion about the play narrative. The carer had been prepared beforehand by the therapist and was supportive of this approach, knowing they could go at a pace that felt manageable for them.

By including a more active contribution from the therapist, the child and carer felt more confident to share a narrative about the many changes and experiences, with a focus on the child's feelings and loss. ●●●

Many of the children seen in the clinical service and within the studies present with indiscriminate and overfamiliar behaviours towards adults. They are avoidant or show disorganised behaviour towards their parent, together with a frequent tendency to approach the therapist rather than their parent. The assessment process will have indicated whether the child often turns to other adults so that using a more direct approach with the child can be considered and used where appropriate.

Later sessions of the intervention commonly use these approaches, once the child has established a preference and greater emotional reliance on the parent. The parent and child can then be supported to find ways to maintain their closer relationship in the presence of others. They can also be supported to adapt to more varied situations, similar to ones in their wider family and network. This also tests the child's capacity to maintain the emotional and behavioural connection with the parent, and the therapist can help the child to discriminate how they relate to different adults simultaneously.

CASE STUDY O

Child O was aged 2 and a half years. As this intervention progressed, the therapist spoke directly to the child to try and clarify his communication about his choices and wishes and encouraged him to signal these more clearly. It also helped highlight O's signals for his parent who missed many of his cues and generally was very directive. The therapist made brief comments to clarify the child's interest to help progress the play but then stood back to show support for the parent's response to their child. ●●●

There are children who experience separation anxiety or who have developed an anxious ambivalent style of relating to their parent. The therapist's relationship with the child needs to be carefully negotiated to introduce more direct contact with the child over time. This is more effective once the parent has gained some insight into the underlying anxiety the child feels. The parent could also become more aware of the possible mixed messages they give to their child about being more autonomous, e.g. frequently communicating to the child that they must try to do things by themselves and inconsistently offering help/support.

Direct approaches from therapist to child:

- Short comments to the child to help contain them in the moment, e.g. 'Daddy is thinking of you', if the child finds it hard to share attention when their parent is talking and the parent is unable to divide their attention.
- Referencing possible underlying emotions such as anger or worry in the child, especially if there are only fleeting expressions and it is difficult for the parent to notice as it is anxiety provoking for them, e.g. 'You are wanting someone to help... I think you need Mummy'.
- Articulating an observed need of the child, e.g. 'I think that might have hurt when you tripped...'
- Prompts to the child to communicate or interact with their parent such as 'Come and show Mummy where your knee hurts' or 'Bring the toy over, Mummy can help', 'You look like you need a hug from Daddy'.
- Commenting on specific stressors/traumatic events through supporting the child with symbolic play or reading a book with a related theme, alongside the parent, e.g. commenting on the actions in the play: 'The children are fighting, hungry/the parents are cross with each other'.
- Facilitating the play to continue by passing a toy to the child, bringing objects nearer, when the interaction is fragile and liable to breakdown rapidly between parent and child.

Figure 5.4 Examples of direct approaches from the therapist to the child

When the parent has begun to make some changes in their approach (with more active attempts to help the child) and shows that they are available when needed, they can remain responsive and emotionally available to the child, even when the therapist is offering direct support to the child. Talking to the parent and being explicit about what the therapist will do, and what role the parent maintains, also helps to support the direct work and does not undermine the progress in the relationship between parent and child. For example, if the child becomes distressed, the therapist may articulate this but will support the child to seek out the parent for comfort.

CASE STUDY P

Child P, aged 3 and a half years, presented initially with severe separation difficulties and could not respond to the therapist at all. As the intervention progressed and changes were seen in the parent–child relationship, the therapist checked with mother before offering P help with a toy. She accepted this for a short period before returning to her parent. With sensitive repetition, she gradually built confidence in managing to relate to the therapist and parent at the same time. ●●●

2 Reflective discussion and direct work with parents

The intervention approach includes direct work with the parent and is tailored to support their well-being, emotional regulation and reflective functioning. This helps them to develop insight into their child's emotional needs and into their own responses and mental states.

The next section will:

- explore general considerations about the context for the focused parent work
- briefly describe the concepts of reflective functioning or mind-mindedness, which provide a framework related to a parent's capacity to think about and respond to their child's emotional states
- look at examples of using the intervention to promote and develop this further.

THE CONTEXT FOR THE FOCUSED PARENT WORK

Communicating respect and empathy

From the start of the assessment the therapist is highly attuned to the parent's emotional well-being and mental states (hopes, anxieties, unresolved feelings, motivations, etc.) and their capacity to regulate and reflect on these. It is essential that the therapist shows an open, respectful and empathic response to the parent's view and feelings; this is of central importance to the therapist understanding both the parent's experience as well as that of their child, and the relationship between them.

Most parents feel very sensitive when their role and relationship with their child is focused on, often with a sense that they are 'under scrutiny' or being judged. Even in everyday life, parents may feel upset or annoyed if family or members of the public make comments about their parenting or refer to their child's behaviour as an indication of poor or misguided parenting. Special care is needed for parents who may have already had a lifetime of adversity and experienced chronic low self-esteem, or for parents who have experienced more difficulties since becoming a parent. The work needs to be tailored to supporting, and sometimes gently challenging, them in their parental role, while being mindful that the therapist will have a relatively short period of involvement in their life.

The impact of mental health and past trauma

Some parents are experiencing mental health problems; the most prevalent difficulties being postnatal depression, chronic depression and anxiety. Others may have diagnoses of personality disorder, complex PTSD, psychotic conditions or OCD. Many parents have significant trauma histories involving multiple losses, childhood neglect or abuse, along with current stressors such as marital conflict, domestic abuse, social isolation, immigration problems and poor housing conditions. The work, therefore, needs to include sufficient time to understand how these varied experiences are impacting on the parent's state of mind and mental health in the present, as well as the impact on the relationship with their child and the child's emotional experience. This can raise specific issues and tensions within the clinical work, and particularly the therapeutic relationship, which require ongoing reflection within clinical supervision. For some parents this assessment and intervention is their first contact with a psychologically-based service, whereas for others they may be fully or partially engaged with adult support or mental health services.

Other caregivers and parents who do not have mental health difficulties may experience anxieties from a number of sources, including:

- their pathway to becoming a parent
- worries about their child
- other pressures and life events
- triggers from past experiences in their own childhoods.

Many texts describe the processes affecting parents in different social, family and cultural configurations and contexts (Raphael-Leff, 1991; Hindle & Shulman, 2008).

How past experiences influence attributions

All parents will hold identifications with and representations of their child (and significant others) that influence their emotions, attitudes and actions towards them. These stem from the parent's internalised experience of relationships with their own parents and other key attachment figures/relationships from their past, as well as their more recent history of adolescent and adult relationships. If positive, these can have a helpful impact as the parent can draw on the emotional and psychological resilience they have developed from positive interpersonal experiences. Other parents have internalised distressing, frightening or neglectful experiences that have remained emotionally unresolved. The understanding of these influences on the parent–child relationship was articulated by Selma Fraiberg and has become well known as 'ghosts in the nursery' (Fraiberg, 1994).

With parents who have experienced insecure past relationships, there is often a sense of confusion or mismatch between what the therapist observes and the parent describes. For example, you might hear a strong set of beliefs being used repeatedly that indicate the parent's conflict with particular emotions or vulnerable states. Comments to the child or therapist that include 'stop, don't' or 'never, should' would indicate this confused emotional state, in a defensive attempt to introduce clarity. You will also hear the parent make attributions to the child's behaviour or responses that are misplaced, or distorted to the context and often to the child's developmental level and ability. An example of this could be a parent who experienced abuse in childhood and who was not believed, who reacts angrily to her daughter if she does not behave in the way that the mother has just described to the therapist. The mother feels that she is being shown up as a 'liar' and the child is blamed; the child then experiences an intrusive and incongruous communication from her mother.

Transference and countertransference

These parental unresolved representations and emotional states will also be conveyed through verbal and non-verbal communication in the developing relationship with the therapist. The therapist's own responses to these provide insights into the underlying mental/emotional states of the parent. This is known as transference and countertransference (see Chapter 1). While this may be included in direct work with some parents, it is not a core technique routinely employed. It would be considered in supervision to support the therapist to understand and manage strong emotions that are evoked in the parent and themselves, e.g. fear, despair, rage.

There is wide variety in how much parents share personal information throughout the assessment and intervention.

- Some parents relay detailed accounts of their history from the outset.
- Other parents talk about their own experience as feelings or memories are triggered during the work.
- Some feel unable to think and talk about their past or current emotional experience.

The Adult Attachment Interview research (Main, 2000) also shows that it is the quality of the narratives that indicate whether an individual has been able to think about and process their experience. Therefore, you need to give attention to how a parent is communicating, e.g. reporting distressing events without the associated feelings or with a lack of coherence.

Reflective functioning

This leads onto the theoretical and clinical concepts of reflective functioning developed by Peter Fonagy and colleagues at UCL (Fonagy, Target, Steele & Steele, 1998). They define 'reflective functioning' as:

> *'the capacity to understand that one's own or another's behaviours are linked in meaningful ways to underlying mental states, to feelings, wishes, thoughts and desires'.*

Turning to the parenting role specifically, Arietta Slade refers to their work and the importance of:

> *'the parent's capacity to reflect upon the child's internal experience... so crucial to the development of a secure attachment and to a range of other developmental outcomes.'* (Slade, 2005)

Slade and Fonagy have commented on the link between reflective functioning and containment (Bion, 1962b) and that these have a function on both a mental as well as a behavioural level. This is helpful as it relates directly to the simultaneous need for the parent to both show understanding of the child's emotional needs and to demonstrate that they are able to manage it on a practical, visible level. In therapeutic work we see some parents being more skilled at mirroring their child's emotions but are less able to act in a parental role to help the child master the feelings; other parents may do the opposite and respond in a predictable, stable way to the behaviour without acknowledging the emotions of the child.

A parent's varied insight into how their own emotional states and behaviour may affect their child brings significant challenges to the clinical parent–child work. It requires sensitive timing and pacing within the therapeutic process. It may be that a parent becomes more aware of the emotional impact of their state of mind on their baby as they themselves are recovering from a period of depression or a particularly stressful time when they had been preoccupied. This can cause the parent a great deal of distress with further anxiety and guilt. With the therapist's containment of this upset, as well as a communication of hope for the relationship and the child's well-being, this can be worked with and resolved to some degree. It reflects the reality that there are difficult issues to address as well as the potential for positive change. It is important that the therapist does not just exclusively offer reassurance to the parent about the more difficult time that the parent and child have lived through: they can use this as an opportunity to think about both of their experiences, which reinforces the importance of their relationship.

Helping the parent to increase their insight into their own and their child's thoughts and feelings is known to reduce stress levels. This is because the parent's greater understanding of the child's responses or behaviour leads to a greater sense of coping or mastery (McMahon & Meins, 2012). However, this work needs to progress at a pace that feels manageable on an emotional and practical level for the parent. This ensures benefits for the relationship, as well as the parent and child individually.

A range of approaches should be considered as some parents' mental states and stress levels can fluctuate rapidly and may be triggered by attending to the child's emotional cues differently, or by shifts in the relationship. Timing needs to be thought about carefully when addressing:

- the parent's mindset towards the child in relation to specific misattributions
- identifications of the child with self/others
- role reversal.

This is because these are likely to be connected to the parent's past unresolved traumas.

TECHNIQUES WITH PARENTS

A range of different techniques and approaches with the parent are needed, which are used in conjunction with the live parent–child work. They have been described as separate techniques below although they are often used in conjunction with each other in clinical work.

1. Parents' reflections on parent–child interactions within the live work

All parents and caregivers experience strong emotions at times when interacting with their baby or young child. This early period of the child's development can stir up powerful feelings (positive, negative, vulnerable, etc.). Initially, these feelings may be outside of the adult's consciousness, especially those who have unresolved past stress and trauma.

Whether in the home or other settings, natural interactions occur between parents and children and you will observe and experience these with them moment to moment. You may see positive cycles of interaction, or fleeting moments of shared interest and pleasure, that can be enjoyed and acknowledged between child and parent through gestures or words. Equally there may be great difficulty for some parents and children in managing more positive or intimate moments; it can seem that these are being avoided or 'lost' in a second, or that the parent and child are unable to 'trust' that this kind of experience can be part of their relationship for a variety of reasons.

You may witness distorted, disjointed and disturbing interactions that have a very negative or confusing quality. These can be painful to experience for all involved. Sometimes these can be moments when the therapist receives a greater force of emotional impact than the parent, or child, appears to be in touch with. The therapist themself may be brought into these interactions by the parent or child. Therefore they need to be sensitive to what role they may be being given and how to respond to this at the time, and to be able to record this for later reflection. For example, a parent may, in an outwardly neutral way, comment to their toddler that the therapist is more able to help the child than they are as a parent. They might direct the child to be closer to the therapist, while distancing themselves in the room, or if at home even leaving the room itself.

The different kinds of micro-interactions and their associated emotional qualities are infinite in their individuality and meaning for parent–child dyads. The general approaches of reflecting with parents in the 'live work' on specific moments with their child can support their understanding of the child's underlying emotional states, motivations and attachment needs.

The following case studies illustrate how the therapist may note the responses between child and parent, along with an awareness of the possible sub-script(s) from both. The therapist may then respond at the time, first observing and then subsequently noting when the same pattern of interaction arises. This clinical judgement is based on issues including the therapeutic engagement, timing within the session, and whether there have been previous discussions about this aspect of the relationship that can be linked to helpfully.

In trying to engage the parent's thoughts about their child's particular action or response to them, one can weave in comments about the parent's contribution. It is more straightforward to draw on a positive example of something that the parent has done that has elicited a positive response from the child (but which has often gone unnoticed by the parent until articulated out loud by the therapist). But it's necessary to think sensitively about situations where the interaction has disrupted and may be spiralling into negative cycles due to automatic sub-conscious triggers.

Addressing the triggers for more negative reactions from the parent is described further in the next section. It may be more appropriate to discuss this after the child's more immediate needs have been attended to and the dyad has had the opportunity to experience the recovery of their interaction or to create a new beginning: 'an interactive repair' (Tronick, 1989).

However the appropriateness and timing of a more exploratory discussion with the parent is considered in relation to each clinical picture, it may be that it is better to leave it to a later time in the intervention. In some cases it may not be raised directly, depending on the parent's mental state and what they wish to bring into the work. Another reason for staying within the moment is that it can be very helpful for the parent to reflect on what has just been experienced with their child, along with the specific emotions and thoughts that it raises for them. These may include a sense of joy, but the parent may also experience sadness and guilt as they become aware of how little they have been engaged with their child in the way that has just been experienced. It also creates the chance to hear what intentions a parent attributes to their child's behaviour. These can be discussed more at the time and/or in a later conversation.

The following case studies have been created to give a snapshot of the clinical approach, where the therapist intervenes with comments, support and suggestions as to how the parent might notice and/or respond to their child in a different way.

CASE STUDY Q

Child Q, aged 6 months, lived with his mother, who had been in care herself and had a history of self-harm. Mum had an older child who was now adopted. Q's mum became more in touch with her own worry and distress during the intervention. She became quite upset in response to any perceived signs that her baby might not need her. She would then quickly become frustrated with her son and would make critical remarks about him. The therapist talked with mum about the negative attributions in one to one discussion. In the joint live work, the therapist continued to engage mum to consider the underlying emotional states of her baby, e.g. when he needed to down-regulate, requiring comfort despite not crying. This helped the mother to remain involved with her baby in a less intrusive way, offering her baby attention and comfort. The therapist could then reinforce the positive response from the baby when he was comforted and showing interest in his mother and play. ●●●

CASE STUDY R

Child R was a 14-month-old toddler. She had presented as highly avoidant in the assessment but made some changes early on during the intervention in response to mum's capacity to reach out to her more. Mum became more hopeful as the therapist pointed out R's responses to her. This increased dependence on her created some tension, and she could acknowledge the greater demands on her as a result. She had held strong beliefs that her daughter was not interested in her and that she was better free to roam, needing little input from her mother. Mum responded to the help from the therapist to think how she could be involved in joint play with her daughter and also cope with the moments when R wanted to be more autonomous. ●●●

CASE STUDY S

Child S was 2 and a half years old. Following a traumatic incident when S witnessed domestic abuse, Child S had become anxious, angry and controlling, which her mother found very difficult to reflect on. During sessions mum would feel overwhelmed easily, become directive herself, and a negative cycle would ensue. At these moments of tension, the therapist would introduce ideas about what feelings were present for them both. Anger was a difficult emotion for mum to acknowledge as she also felt so guilty that the child had been frightened by the incident. Therefore, the therapist reflected on these mixed emotions, articulating the anger both mum and child clearly felt at times. Mum began to respond to the therapy space by slowing down and being more reflective herself, naming feelings for her child which contained rather than instructed her behaviour. ●●●

2. Explore attributions to, and identifications with, the child from the 'live' work

This section describes an approach which involves the parent on a one to one basis to explore conflicting and/or intense emotions that arise during the parent–child work. It is important to consider what may be included in this part of the work as it could be mistaken for discussing the history of the adult's childhood or other specific distressing/traumatic events. Although this may be a component of some discussions with parents (where the adult has raised memories that are on their mind, or which have been triggered by an emotional experience they have had with their baby/child) it is more usually a time when the parent reflects on feelings or responses they have become aware of currently that cause them distress and anxiety.

We are led by the pace and depth to which the adult of the dyad wishes to share and/or access narratives of their own experience before and since becoming a parent. Careful thought needs to be given within supervision and case reviews to what discussion and exploration of the adult's personal history is addressed in these sessions, even when they have already told the therapist a great deal about their past and current stressors. Therapists should be aware that some parents need to 'tell all' as a way of trying to rid themselves of the experiences that are so painful, but not in a manner that lends itself to any thought and digestion. Some individuals say too much too quickly and this should not be confused with greater self-awareness and a wish to explore issues in more depth. This may be far from what is possible or helpful to the individual's mental state and coping mechanisms. The parents' past experiences may cause them confusion and lead them to repeat negative cycles in their relationship with their young child – the 'ghosts in the nursery'. Therefore, careful consideration is given to the inclusion, or omission, of links with the parent's own personal history which you could hypothesise are relevant to the parent's views and responses to their child.

As well as specific remembered events and emotions, the therapist may talk with the parent about the feelings that arise at a specific moment. They may also talk about how they wish to manage them differently (where this is of relevance to the adult and important for the parent–child relationship). It may be that the discussions centre more on issues that have occurred in the live parent–child work where the therapist has seen the difficulty for the parent when the child shows particular needs or heightened emotional states. Therefore it may be more appropriate to talk with, and empathise about, how challenging this is and to think about how the parent may want to respond so that it reduces the impact on the dyad. The parent can then feel more confident in their capacity to cope and to stop repeating difficult moments.

There may be circumstances when the parent brings strongly expressed emotions into the relationship with the therapist, and the contact and support offered is experienced in a negative or persecutory way. In these instances the therapist needs to bring this to their own supervision for further thought and recommendations about how to respond to the parent. This is common in all therapies to different degrees and will arise throughout the therapy process. It often needs addressing more directly if it begins to compromise the engagement of the parent–child work, evidenced in cancelled appointments or repeated dismissive or negative comments.

The therapist needs to be mindful that this may have an impact on the relationships within the network, especially if the parent has a period of time when they feel negatively towards the therapist delivering the intervention.

The following case studies illustrate how this work may be integrated within the intervention and be addressed in some of the different ways described. The scenarios are by no means exhaustive.

CASE STUDY T

Child T was aged 6 months. After a period of parent–child work, T's Mum needed one to one time with the therapist in some later sessions of the intervention to think about her own distress. She had talked about the fact that, when she cried, it had no effect on her baby and left her feeling uncared for. Mum seemed unaware of the distorted nature of her expectation of her baby. When she went on to explore memories of her childhood, she made links to her own mother. Maternal grandmother had been very unavailable to her through alcohol misuse, depression and several separations, when mum had been taken into care. She became able to think more about her own baby's vulnerability once she had time to reflect on her own position as a child and the experiences she had had to manage too much by herself. ●●●

CASE STUDY U

Child U was aged 12 months. In the parent–child live work, mum had spoken of her anxiety about how her child's behaviour had been affected by her episode of post-natal depression. She became more reflective about the link with her own childhood in one to one sessions, and the distant relationship she had experienced with her own mother. It was distressing when she considered her own child's emotional and physical avoidance of her in recent months. Painful feelings of not being 'good enough' came alive in the work in the joint sessions and she needed help to recognise and contain these so she could be proactive in sharing ideas and experiences with her child. ●●●

CASE STUDY V

Child V was aged 11 months. Mother found it difficult to attribute any emotional states or vulnerability to her child, who had adapted by being overly independent. She would reframe any upset in her child as being due to physical causes. As the intervention progressed she began to express feelings about wishing to hurt her child. She started to reflect on the parallels with her own early childhood when her parents had been unavailable and experiencing mental health problems themselves. Her anger at the therapist's unavailability in between sessions could be articulated and thought about. This helped her to feel more contained and begin to tolerate feelings of vulnerability in herself and her baby. ●●●

3. Review specific cycles of interaction to reinforce strengths and address 'stuck' patterns

As conversations with parents unfold, the therapist gradually develops a sense of the degree to which a parent may be ready to explore the past drivers and coping mechanisms that are influencing their everyday responses and actions within their parenting. Some parents are not ready or do not wish to unpick this in more detail; in these circumstances you need to respect this and find other ways to help them and their child to be freed up from painful 'stuck' cycles.

One helpful approach is to create time with parents to focus on:

- specific situations they have highlighted as problematic, or
- repeating patterns of interaction that have been discussed as they have arisen in previous sessions (both positive and/or negative).

It is helpful to start with an informal review of positive cycles. This begins the process of thinking about the reciprocal and spiral nature of interactions that build on one another. Therapists used a number of different ways to talk about and illustrate this with parents' input and preferences, including:

- specific themed handouts developed in the study (available via the weblink given on page 16 of the Introduction)
- visual materials
- relevant video clips (YouTube)
- their own videos if taken in the assessment.

When moving on to think about more difficult and maladaptive cycles, it is prefaced with how well the parent is doing in a general way, acknowledging the effort they are making in trying to create positive change for their child. However, there can be relief in naming the more difficult areas, with the hope that there is a solution. At the right time many parents are able to join in a discussion that explores both the child's contribution to the relationship along with their own. Clearly this is done with sensitivity and attunement to the pace at which the parent can think through what has happened between them and their child. This is especially the case if the interactions are likely to be associated with painful past events, e.g. when the parent was less available due to mental or physical ill health, or exposure to domestic violence.

The following case study is an example of a parent who was not ready to discuss any of their own childhood history.

CASE STUDY W

Child W was aged 8 months. W's mother became quickly overwhelmed with frustration when her baby did not respond to her efforts to engage or comfort them. Her baby was withdrawn and quiet in general and did not initiate any interaction with mum. She found any reflective discussion of what was happening difficult. However, she started to respond to the therapist giving her very immediate support and encouragement to persist with her baby at the first sign of tension in the interaction. She went on to make use of **Handout 8: Positive cycles** midway through the intervention. This was the start of her being able to talk more easily about the relationship with her baby. ●●●

4. Psychoeducation: infant/child development and emotional regulation

Many approaches in parent–child therapy incorporate some form of information sharing with parents (which Selma Fraiberg originally described as 'developmental guidance'). The parents' experience of the parenting they had received was extremely variable, often with significant gaps in ordinary and consistent experience of available and supportive parental figures. As well as the emotional impact from the patchy or inadequate care they received, the therapist considers what gaps there may be in their knowledge of what babies and young children generally need to support their development and social–emotional well-being.

For other parents who have experienced a greater sense of security in their childhoods but who have received a child into their family through adoption or kinship care, there can be other challenges with caring for a child who has experienced trauma and loss. This adds to the difficulty in not having the early, shared history of infancy. For example, it can be particularly hard for those who adopt a child who is in the toddler phase of pushing for independence; the foundations of dependence will not yet have been laid and this can be hard to address when the child has established specific defences.

Parents' existing knowledge and belief systems about what young children require from their parents is often revealed through the discussions in the assessment about the child's presentation and the expectations that the parent has of the child. A commonly heard view is that it is better to leave a distressed child on their own to recover, or they may become 'spoiled'. Other beliefs include how independent a young child should be, and there are many more. It is useful to listen out for the statements that include the word 'should' as these are often the ones that denote strongly held and possibly intractable beliefs.

If it is difficult to extend a conversation with parents about their beliefs regarding their child or the relationship if they are too preoccupied or not able to be reflective; a useful starting point can be to introduce a handout. **Handout 1: Commonly held beliefs about babies and children** expresses a range of beliefs about childhood/children's needs, including those that might be considered to be 'myths'. Parents could talk through their responses to them, often evoking other lines of thought that had not previously been expressed. For example, one parent did not agree with most of the 'beliefs' noted on the handout, but it prompted her to reflect on her feeling that her baby son was not 'clingy enough' and had developed a prematurely independent way of being. She then became in touch with her sadness about this. Specific handouts have been created to reflect the different stages of development to resonate with the parent's own child, i.e. one for the infant period and another for the toddler stage.

A range of resources were developed and others were collated from widely available sources to help provide information and thought about aspects of a baby's/young child's changing needs over time, integrating the contribution made by the caregiving (parent–child) environment. Tailored to the individual parent(s), and being mindful of the influences from extended family members, specific video, visual and/or written materials were shared with the parent in the first instance, which they sometimes passed on to other key figures in the family or network.

The following case studies show how these resources can be used variably to match the needs of the individual situation.

CASE STUDY X

Child X was aged 14 months. This toddler's mother asked to watch the video of herself and her child playing in the assessment period. This raised questions for her about the impact of her depression, and she and the therapist went on to look at some clips from the strange situation videos and still face experiments. Mother found these emotionally hard to watch on the one hand, reflecting how she felt she had had a 'still face' herself for a period. However, she felt that it gave her a framework for understanding what had happened for her and her child. This seemed to help the mother to think through the experience on an emotional and cognitive level, and she spoke of it making her feel less alone with the experience. ●●●

CASE STUDY Y

Child Y was aged 3. Y had been injured in a car accident as a baby. Mother was an experienced parent but had been overwhelmed by guilt and found it impossible to reflect on her child's feelings and to set reasonable and appropriate boundaries for her daughter. Mum wanted to look through the written resources and video clips relating to attachment concepts. For her, this was a gentle way of getting in touch with her own knowledge and to start to think about the feelings underlying a child's behaviour, and the role of the parent to respond and contain them. ●●●

5. Individual 'Activity template' for the child and parent

In a number of clinical situations that used the psychoeducation approach described above, the parents also benefited from individualised resources. These resources described specific elements of the interaction and the child's needs that had been previously identified in the assessment. These resources are referred to as the 'Activity templates' because they give practical suggestions for ways in which the parent might respond to or engage in activity with their child, e.g. how to introduce play at bathtime when their child finds this transition hard to manage. Two examples (Activity template A and Activity template B) can be accessed via the link provided on page 16 of the Introduction.

Activity templates were first developed when running the pilot study in 2010. In order to give the family a record or 'crib' sheet of the ideas that had been discussed and recommended, the Activity templates were trialled in the clinical service, each one created individually for the child and parent. They articulated suggestions for joint activities that were graded to the child/parent relationship at that stage and time. They included specific situations when the child might need a particular attuned response from the parent, e.g. when in the presence of strangers, at goodbyes and reunions.

In light of the positive response from parents (and professionals), use of the Activity templates continued. They were developed further so that they became part of interventions where the parent found it helpful to approach emotionally-loaded topics with practical tangible knowledge and learning. With the reality that many families experience chronic and new stressors in their everyday life, these templates gave some sense of continuity and prompts to the parents in between sessions.

The Activity templates were designed to be user-friendly for parents who were more focused on the concrete aspects of their parenting and their child's behaviour. They provided another means of introducing themes of the child's emotional and mental states and what they required from their parent in turn.

The term 'Activity' was broad and ranged from play ideas and everyday activities, such as mealtimes, to more general interactions, such as setting boundaries, comforting when hurt or talking about specific situations with the child. They could include:

- ideas of ways to manage specific presenting difficulties
- activities to promote underlying needs
- ways of supporting the child with individual stressors
- new play ideas to help shift patterns of interacting by introducing a new dynamic.

It was useful to return to the Activity templates in clinical sessions, to review progress and discuss challenges when trying to complete these activities. They could also be shared with others, for example nursery staff, social workers, or contact workers in a variety of ways and contexts, e.g. the activity ideas might focus on support around transitions, e.g. between home and nursery.

Below is a description of when an Activity template was used within the intervention.

CASE STUDY Z

Child Z was aged 3 and a half years. This child and mother had developed some distorted patterns of relating to one another, though we had also identified positive interactions in the assessment that we could feed back. Mother was keen to try new ways of interacting with her child but found reflective discussion very difficult, requiring a lot of repetition in the parent–child 'live' work to sustain any change. The Activity template created for them helped to support the mother to hold on to the ideas and put them into practice.

When mum referred to difficult behaviours that occurred in between sessions, the therapist could refer back to the different topics covered on the Activity template which helped her to make the connection between different behaviours. It included ideas for:

- how the mother could maintain a connection with her child while they were engaged in separate activities (e.g. child playing and mum doing other tasks)
- new ways of playing together that supported new interaction patterns
- activities to try when interactions started to become difficult and to prevent negative cycles
- ways of setting boundaries in an age-appropriate way that help a child to succeed (as the mother could have very high expectations)
- ideas for talking to the child about the impending arrival of a new sibling. ●●●

6. Handouts and homework sheets

The handouts and homework sheets can be included in the intervention sessions with parents if it is felt they will be helpful. For many families they are not appropriate, as they could be experienced as pressurising, inaccessible or condescending. Therefore the decision to incorporate this element of the intervention is made on a case by case basis and can be informed by the parents' response to the initial assessment. General handouts on a range of themes were created and introduced flexibly (as described in more detail in Chapter 6). These are all available via the online link on page 16 of the Introduction. They can be adapted in different services for their populations as appropriate.

For those families who engaged with some of the early written and visual materials, Homework sheets might be introduced. This gave parents the chance to have a focused and more structured way of thinking about their child's development and needs. The parent could record their responses to a given situation (e.g. responding when their child was distressed), which were then reviewed in subsequent face to face intervention sessions. Flexibility around integrating them in interventions was important because, for many families, external life events were occurring on a frequent basis, along with fluctuating changes in their own mental or physical health. This meant that parents needed space to talk about this first. Sessions would then focus predominantly on how this was observably affecting the relationship and the child in the moment, and reflections on the Homework sheets could be brought back later.

The Homework sheets were largely visual; a range of adult, baby and child graphics of facial expressions or actions were created so that the sheet could be made individual to the family. For example, if a father was the primary caregiver and the child was of toddler age or above, the Homework sheet would be produced accordingly. Most of them only required that a tick or graphic was linked to a theme or relational activity that was the focus at that time. For example, the parent would choose the picture of a child that was most in line with their own baby at moments being discussed. Therefore there was little or no demand for parents to write anything, but this was always an option and some parents used this opportunity to capture their thoughts and feelings. In situations when parents did not complete the Homework sheets, they sometimes described thinking about the 'homework' task while a situation with their child was occurring at home. During the session it was then possible to discuss the different situations that had occurred during the week and how it related to the parent–child 'live' work. At times it was helpful to complete the Homework sheet in the session as a reflective tool and record.

Examples below illustrate using the Homework sheets and Activity templates.

CASE STUDY AA

Child AA was aged 18 months. AA's father found it hard to recognise and accept a range of emotions in his child. With support, he began to identify and name emotions which made him better able to support his child in managing these. The Homework sheets allowed him to see his role in maintaining this outside of the sessions. This supported him to think about his and his child's emotional experience during busy everyday situations that occurred, e.g. breakfast time in a busy household, nursery drop off, playing, and conflicts with older siblings. ●●●

CASE STUDY BB

Child BB was aged 4 months. Although BB's teenage mother lacked confidence and found written work difficult, she completed the Homework sheet every week. She found the practical task a helpful link between sessions, as well as having something to share at the beginning of the next meeting. Her emotional vocabulary was limited so the visual way to record basic emotions on a scale allowed for more discussion around her own, and her baby's, emotional experience. ●●●

CASE STUDY CC

This example describes the use of an Activity template outside of intervention sessions.

Child CC was aged 3 years. She had become looked after and so initially the Activity template was written for her birth mother to use during contact sessions. Contact sessions were difficult for both this young girl and her mother as they were unable to engage in any activities together. The child had been diagnosed with ASD, and the behaviours associated with this seemed especially marked during contact sessions, which mum found hard to manage. The Activity template gave simple ideas of modifying activities to make it easier for both child and parent to engage, and gave concrete ways for mother to support her in contact. This was discussed with the mother and social worker together and prompted new approaches to be introduced in contact sessions, e.g. suggestions for the types of toys the contact team could make available and different ways that mother could follow her daughter's lead.

In addition to the direct work with mum, the Activity template was also shared with the contact worker and there was a phone consultation to think about ways for the contact worker to support the activities and relationship. The contact worker had also found it hard to engage with this child and the ideas were useful for her to consider how she could facilitate CC's engagement and support her emotionally.

The Activity template was shared with the foster carer who in turn suggested that the nursery had a copy as they had been struggling with her. This led to a phone conversation between the therapist and the child's nursery key worker as several of the themes were relevant to her time there and activities were adapted for the nursery setting. This was useful as, until then, the nursery had understood her presentation primarily through consideration of her ASD diagnosis. The conversation regarding the individualised Activity template prompted more thought about the contribution of her early experiences of neglect to her current social-emotional needs. ●●●

Ending sessions of intervention

As with all therapeutic approaches, the final sessions require careful thought. The client (in this clinical approach this includes both child and parent(s), and network to an extent) should have an ending that:

- recognises the work, effort and progress they have made
- acknowledges the loss of the therapeutic relationship and any anxiety about whether the changes can be sustained and held onto.

The therapist also has to contain these feelings and concerns, which may include some of their own anxiety, especially when working with vulnerable families. There are often ongoing challenges that may arise from the families' past or current situational stressors; these may impinge on and threaten some newly formed and developing changes. In interventions that are time-limited, as is the case with the SUSI model, the parents can feel relief at the start of the work that there is an ending in sight in the short- to medium-term. Alongside this, the emotional significance of the relationship with the therapist develops, for the parent and to a lesser degree for the child, as the intervention progresses.

It is important therefore that the ending phase is discussed in supervision or case reviews, not only to address the direct work involved with the parent and child but to think about how this will impact on the wider system. Planning and discussions around this with partner agencies and the parents are critical in helping the transition for the family. They are also needed to consider options about whether other forms of support may be needed or not, along with the timeframe in which these could be most beneficial. In this phase, the network may also need to work more closely, so that the anxiety felt by the family (or possibly in parts of the network) is not acted out in a way that either idealises or rubbishes the clinical work coming to an end.

The system of follow-up review appointments, delivered in the study model, can also be translated into a clinical service. It has many advantages in helping to reinforce and support the progress made. In situations where the intervention was effectively a 'treatment trial', the review can help inform thoughts about alternative packages of care/support if there was less positive change at the end of the intervention. For the majority of families, the review carried out a month or so after the intervention finished, and then six months later, proved supportive in providing a space to continue to reflect on their relationship and the child's needs, and to consider the next developmental phase.

Tailoring the intervention

This early help is vital – I had a baby placed with me who couldn't make an attachment. He used to wriggle and squirm to free himself and rock back and forwards. The support helped me to understand him and with suggestions and advice, and with time and patience, he was able to trust me.

FOSTER PARENT

The rationale of a tailored approach to the intervention has been explored already (see Introduction and Chapter 2). The focus below is on examples which show how the intervention can be delivered to parents whose families are differently constituted and who have children of varying ages and developmental stages. Thought will then be given to some variations in the contextual base that families in different clinical populations may belong to, and the influences, demands and structures of different inter-agency pathways. Adaptations to the direct work and liaison with professionals are described in 'Tailoring to different targeted populations' on page 138.

Tailoring intervention to the families

In this chapter the stages of clinical work have been described, along with the techniques in the initial and central sessions that constitute the core approaches of the intervention. The clinical approaches have been split into two main categories which address:

1. **parent-child 'live' work**, along with techniques that can be used to support change in the parent–child relationship
2. **reflective work with the parent**, in practice this often co-occurs with the live work (as illustrated by some of the clinical case studies).

In order to provide clear descriptions of the component parts of these core approaches, it has been necessary to separate them out in an artificial way; this would not be seen so distinctly in direct clinical practice. Figures 5.5. and 5.6 on pages 135 and 136 illustrate how the clinical approaches can come together and provide an integrated treatment for each family.

- Mother with 3-year-old boy.
- Mum had a diagnosis of unstable personality disorder, somatising symptoms, labile moods and high expressed emotion.
- Father became engaged and contributed to assessment, and although working full-time he joined in discussion with therapist.
- There was conflict in the marriage.

↓

- Child was over-active, aggressive, destructive, and clingy towards mum.
- Children didn't want to play with him.

↓

- Feedback with both mother and father.
- Father expressed worry that the child would be labelled. Mother agreed to the intervention.

↓

- Intervention began in the home but transferred to nursery school setting as the family was in cramped, poor housing and mum was very preoccupied in this environment.

↓

- Initial sessions (1–3) included discussion with mum only who became more emotionally contained.

↓

- Further sessions (4–11) took place in the school setting, which gave focused parent–child work and separate discussion time with mum each session after the child returned to nursery class, to help her reflect on her feelings and relationships.

↓

- Final sessions (12–13), focused on their feelings about ending, and how to continue as a family and included father who wanted to attend.

Figure 5.5 Intervention 1

- Teenage mum and 4-month-old baby.
- Isolated – her only contact was with a FNP worker.

↓

- Baby was very quiet, initiating no interaction.
- Mum lacked the confidence to comfort her and play with her.

↓

- Feedback session with social worker.
- Mother was very quiet but agreed to the intervention, and asked that it took place in a Children's Centre.

↓

Sessions 1–8:

- All parent-child live work, helping support basic interactions.
- Mum could not express any feelings or reflect on her responses and any of her history.

↓

Sessions 9–12:

- Introduced positive and negative cycle resource sheets – she could think of these in the here and now.

↓

Sessions 13–15:

- More parent-child live work and discussion of the relationship in the present.

↓

- Review and review feedback took place with FNP worker.

Figure 5.6 Intervention 2

Revisiting ideas from the feedback stage, it is worth reflecting on the initial discussions with the parent(s) and network about the assessment summary and recommendations. At this point, ideas and insights about the child and/or relationship that were formed during the assessment process are introduced and articulated. There is an attempt to engage with the family to find a shared language when these conversations begin.

The feedback meeting is not the first time that the intervention will have been discussed, so the therapist may already have an idea of the parent's expectations and anxieties about embarking on a greater commitment. During this meeting, conversations can be had about how the intervention may be shaped for the individual family. This brings its own challenges, especially if the parent does not have similar priorities or concerns raised by the clinical team and/or network.

The therapist will consider with the parent(s) how the intervention will begin and what it will focus on. Be aware that the parent could feel threatened if themes and issues that might need to be addressed later are raised too soon. For example, you may have a working hypothesis from the information the parent has shared that they have been affected by recent abuse from domestic violence, as well as emotional neglect and possible abuse in their own childhood, and you have observed that they are unwittingly behaving in a frightening way with their own child now. However, it would be counterproductive to the work if all of this was articulated at the beginning. Instead, it is better to focus on their wish to help their child develop confidence and find ways to manage their feelings and worries, emphasising the central importance of the parent–child relationship.

Some parents have clearly expressed what they would like to work on initially in the intervention, although this is relatively rare. It does, however, serve as an important reminder for professionals not to impose their view about what they feel may be most beneficial. One example of this was with a mother who had shared a great deal of her history during the assessment, including the painful separation from her older son who was in another country; the therapist offered to give time to think further about this, alongside the relationship challenges with her younger son who she cared for now. However, the mother said that she had found it helpful to have been heard in the assessment and she felt ready to focus on the practical and emotional aspects of her relationship with her younger son.

Other parents may express a genuine desire to think about their relationship with their child and the specific issues highlighted by them and the therapist. However, they then struggle with overwhelming preoccupations about their own emotional and mental health. In these instances, the therapist will need to hear and contain the parent's narrative. Simultaneously, they will need to find the timing and space to orientate the parent to think about their child and start to introduce the shared joint focus on the child (described in the section on 'Initial sessions' on page 95).

Figures 5.5 and 5.6 on the previous pages show two illustrations of how the intervention may be delivered. While in both the central focus was on the relationship between parent and child, there were significant differences in the children and the relationship presentations. There were also variations in why and to what degree the parent could consider their contribution in the present and how the past had influenced it. They also show how different approaches were integrated to tailor the intervention in order to support the parent–child dyad, and ultimately the child's well-being and development.

Tailoring to different targeted populations

SUSI was a vital experience for this child: it helped her need to feel understood, nurtured and begin the process of making sense of herself and others within her new home. For the adopters, they felt better equipped as they strived to understand her – they found ways to help her manage her experiences in more positive ways.

ADOPTION SOCIAL WORKER

There are many contextual influences and parameters to consider including the wider family, community and professional networks when getting to know the child and their parents. The groups that made up the clinical cohorts in the SUSI study are used as examples, although they have many variations within themselves. Figures 5.7, 5.8 and 5.9 on the following pages try to capture these while providing different templates to show common characteristics with other clinical or vulnerable populations.

For instance, a young mother who has some community support but is not involved in statutory services, e.g. referred to the Parental Mental Health team or equivalent support service, will have similar lines of communication in relation to a parent–infant/child mental health service, involving network liaison (see Figure 5.8). Two of the groups (LAC and CP) described in Figures 5.7 and 5.9 have some of the most complex inter-agency networks. Together these flowcharts give an overview of how an assessment and therapeutic intervention from the SUSI model can be integrated into different inter-agency pathways to promote greater collaboration.

As described in earlier chapters, clear inter-agency communication helps support the engagement, assessment and feedback with families. Mapping these clear lines of communication at the outset helps parents to know when and how you will liaise and share information with partner agencies. This is important because it helps to avoid drift and delays in assessment or other feedback being shared. In statutory frameworks it also provides a clear mechanism for reports to be made available and for inter-agency liaison to take place in a timely way for key decision-making forums.

All clinical approaches require open and transparent communication with families about information shared with others (outside of specific safeguarding situations). Figures 5.7 to 5.9 illustrate how the professionals are involved across agencies, with the corresponding need to understand one another's roles and working practices. These three examples show the core inter-agency systems for looked after children, a community population and children on a Child Protection Plan.

Issues relating to the dissemination of information can accelerate or hinder work with families depending on how well systems are communicating. Progress of the child–parent dyad in relation to other professionals' input should be held in mind, so that everyone works to support each other's interventions. For example, when Social Care have to make decisions about their assessment of a prospective long-term caregiver (Special Guardian, Adoptive parent), this process can be supported by providing relevant details of the child's needs and the likely demands they will place on the new parent.

The training sessions for the model will include examples of how the direct clinical work is embedded in different professional networks. Thought can be given to the specific context in which the assessment and intervention would be delivered locally.

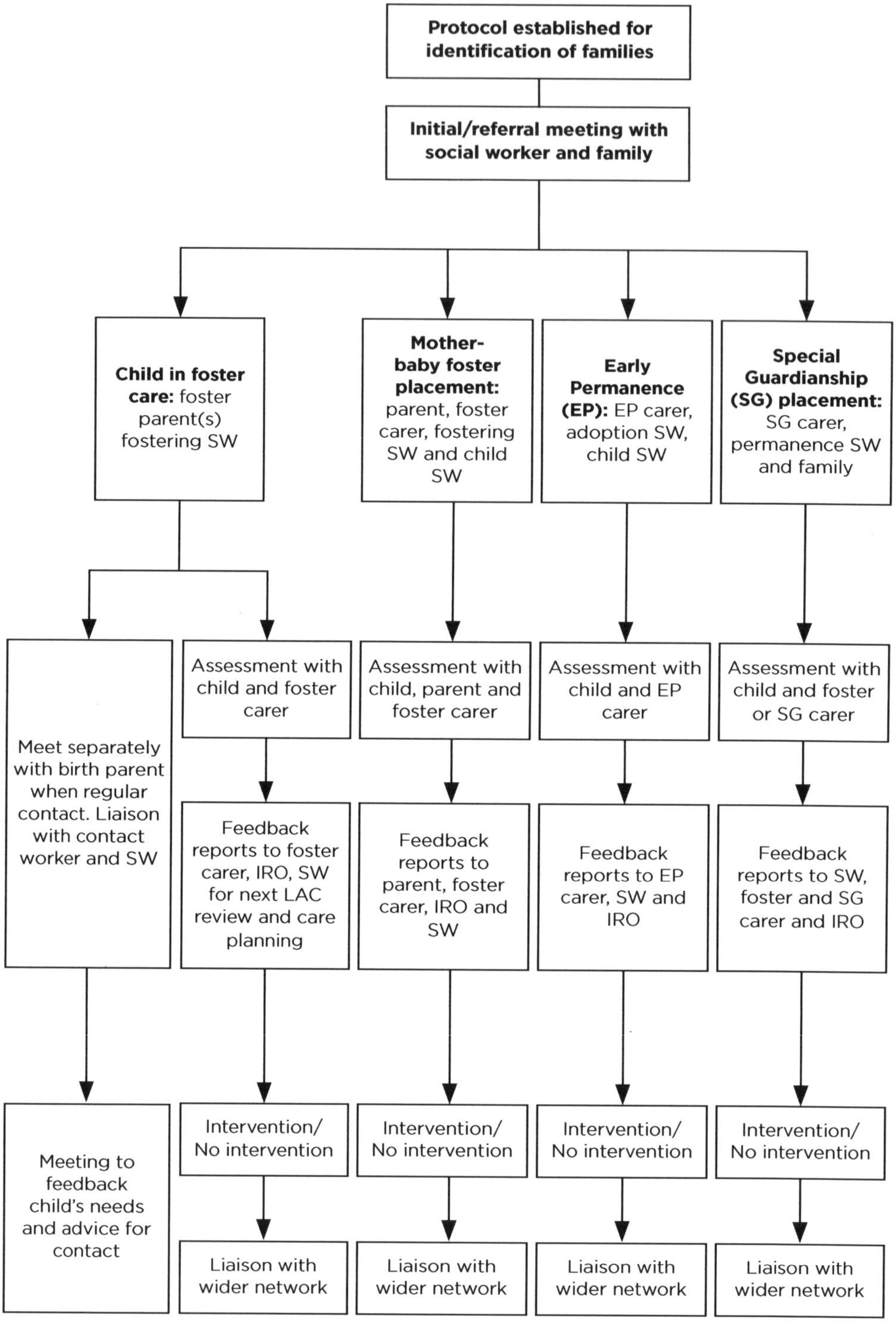

Figure 5.7 The SUSI inter-agency pathway for looked after children

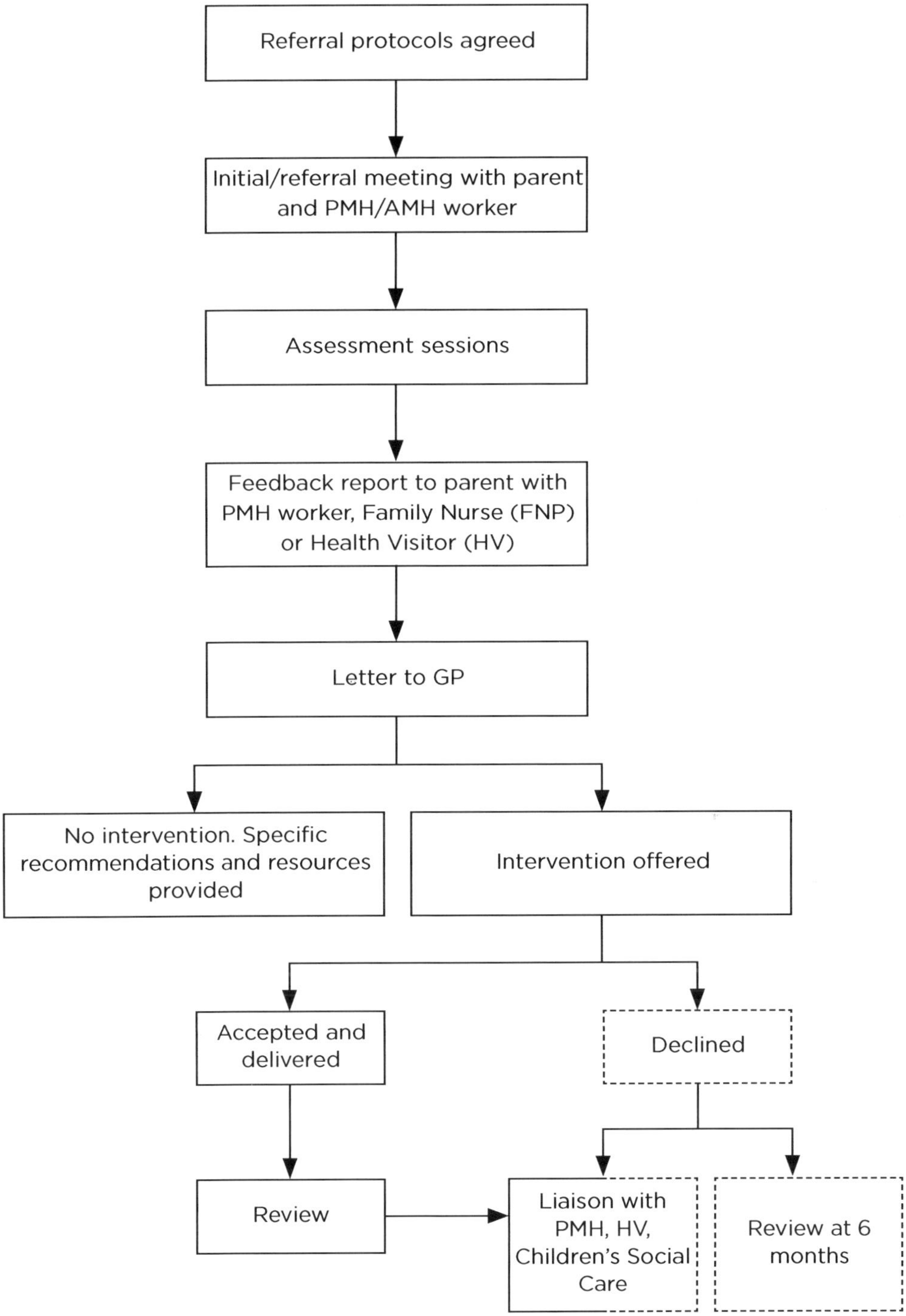

Figure 5.8 The SUSI inter-agency pathway for a community population

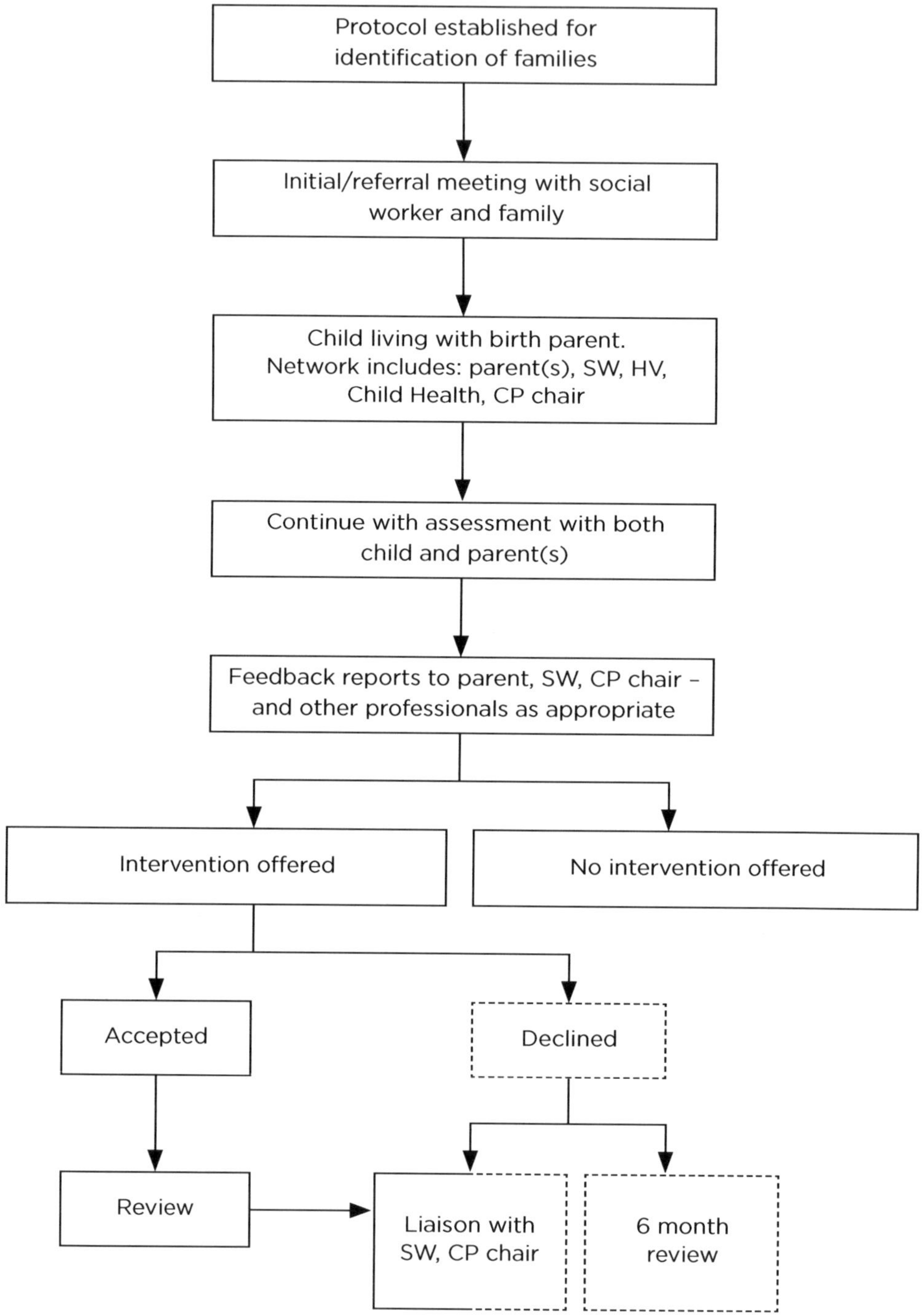

Figure 5.9 The SUSI inter-agency pathway for a child on a Child Protection (CP) Plan

6 Themes for intervention sessions

This chapter sets out the intervention themes that can facilitate a discussion within an individual session. The themes describe key building blocks and dynamics of parent–child relationships that may need support in order to strengthen or create change within them, including:

- the attachment system
- parent's attunement to their child's signals
- autonomy
- joint attention
- shared enjoyment
- emotional regulation
- the reciprocal impact of stress triggers between parent and child.

When delivering a tailored intervention, the themes are incorporated in a flexible way to respond to the needs of the child and family. **Handout 2: Intervention themes** outlines the themes which can be given to and discussed with the parent(s) at the start of the intervention. Initial priorities can be agreed at this stage and then reviewed throughout the work. As before, the term 'parent' is used to describe any primary caregiver to the child, i.e. birth, foster, kinship or adoptive mother or father. One or more parent(s) may be involved in the discussions or direct work relating to the themes.

Intervention themes

All the themes are likely to be relevant for most children and families to varying degrees. The diagram below illustrates that they are not integrated into the work in a specific order. Some will have more resonance than others and may be threaded through several sessions. They have been created as a guide to important topics to be used alongside the therapeutic techniques

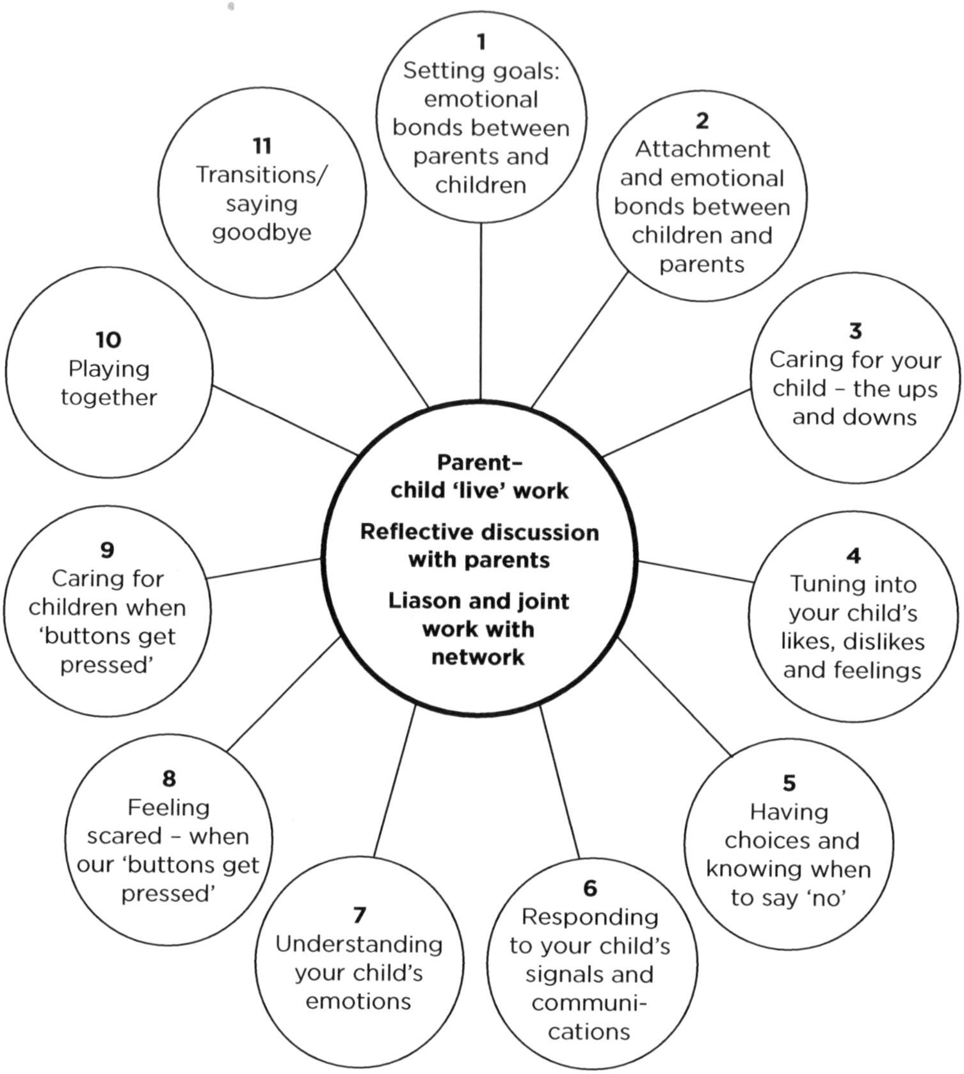

Figure 6.1 Intervention themes

described in Chapter 5. For many families they may serve only as a starting point for conversations. This is because the diversity of each child and family's experience is so great, and discussions and exploration of their individual issues will follow a natural course.

The themes have been outlined under eleven separate headings and have been structured to show the different ways they can be used. There are suggestions for who is involved when discussing the theme (for example, parent only or parent and child) and resources that may be useful. In practice, greater flexibility is needed as some parents will always need to attend with their baby/child or it may be that online resources are used in conjunction with, or are more appropriate and helpful than, the ones devised in the SUSI project.

As described in Chapter 5, finding a shared language with the parent(s) about their child's development and the relationship between them is crucial for building trust and understanding. The suggestions which follow can be adapted and included as appropriate to the developing work between the therapist and family.

Preparation

Prepare a file for each family to hold the resources from the intervention. Include **Handout 2: Intervention themes** which lists the themes that will be talked through in the sessions. Give the message that the work will focus on what is important to them and their child. For example, some themes may be covered at several time-points as needed.

Talk to the parent about the broad 'aims' outlined in **Handout 3: Aims of the SUSI intervention** (which can be adapted to a service's context and target populations) including:

- building secure emotional foundations and confidence in the child
- supporting the child to be an active communicator of thoughts/feelings
- helping the child develop appropriate skills and independence in line with their age and stage
- supporting the child's emotional regulation and positive coping strategies.

Theme 1

Setting goals: emotional bonds between parents and children

RESOURCES

- Individual file for parent(s)
- Assessment report
- Handouts:
  - Handout 1: Commonly held beliefs about babies and children
  - Handout 3: Aims of the SUSI intervention
  - Handout 4: Why is social-emotional development important?
- DVD player or laptop to play video clips
- Access to WiFi

FOCUS

- Individual file for families
- Reflection on assessment – strengths and difficulties
- Discussion of intervention format and content
- Importance of relationships and social-emotional development as a foundation for development

The main focus of this theme is the importance of children having close emotional bonds and relationships with their parents; how the interpersonal experience between parent and child supports a child's healthy development. There is acknowledgement that this involves both the parent and the child taking an active part. It includes the thinking that the strengthening of a child's attachment and social-emotional development forms the foundation for other areas of child development.

There is recognition that both the parent's knowledge of their child and the team's experience will, together, contribute to the work ahead. Existing strengths as well as new ideas are acknowledged as agents for change.

Where possible, the parent(s) discuss this theme in a one to one session without their child.

KEY MESSAGES

- The therapist and parent can reflect on the individual findings of the assessment and any individual goals discussed in the feedback meeting, e.g. strengths of the child, the parent and their relationship, along with difficult dynamics or concerns. The level and detail of this will be informed by the parent's response to the assessment feedback.
- It is essential to acknowledge the contribution that the child makes to the relationship dynamic. For example, how well they signal and communicate their needs. This can link to discussion about how the child's emotional states, e.g. feeling agitated or upset, will evoke feelings in the parent and this may be an opportunity to reflect with the parent about these.
- Introduce the idea that the interpersonal world of the child's relationship with the parent is the critical foundation from which the child will learn and develop. This underpins many areas of development, e.g. growth of attention, cognitive skills, friendships, etc. The intervention is an opportunity to think about the positives as well as the challenges of parenting young babies and children, and of how children develop and grow up.
- We know that the child makes an active contribution to the relationship and that, while the parent's task is to tune into and respond to their child's needs, there can be characteristics of the baby/child that make this more difficult, e.g. being harder to 'read' or soothe. The unique dynamic between child and parent means that 'every child has a different mother/father'.
- General discussions concentrate on recognising when and how children need their parent; and that sometimes the signals can be confusing, making it difficult to understand what the child is trying to communicate and what their needs are. Reflect on the fact that it is normal for young babies and children to be affected by 'strong' emotions which they lack the maturity to manage on their own. These in turn affect the parent who feels these emotions as they are stirred up in them. Recognise the pressures for parents in the 'here and now' as well as from the past and discuss them according to the parent's readiness. Some parents will have explored links between past and present in the assessment phase but for others this will need more time and a different pace.

- **Handout 1: Commonly held beliefs about babies and children** explores the 'beliefs' that parents hold in relation to a child's needs in the early years. This handout includes popular ideas about bringing up babies and children and can be explored to see which resonate for parents from their own family, culture and current community. It is useful as a basis for discussion and to understand the origin of the parent's beliefs. In addition, parents may express a belief in continuing with certain approaches with their child now, or conversely they might not want to repeat the ones they experienced. The common themes within the beliefs include ideas around: crying; giving attention/spoiling; talking to/playing with baby/child; independence/clinging; babies and young children not being able to remember.
- Visual materials may be helpful at this stage, e.g. video clips illustrating the positive influence of the interpersonal social relationship between parent and child.

TRANSITION TO NEXT SESSION/HOMEWORK

This will be included on an individual basis. Where appropriate and helpful, the therapist may suggest other resources that a parent could read or watch before the next session.

Theme 2

Attachment and emotional bonds between children and parents

RESOURCES

- Handouts:
  - Handout 5: To and fro of the parent-child relationship
  - Handout 6: What are attachment behaviours?
  - Handout 7: Attachment and managing emotions
  - Handout 8: Positive cycles
  - Handout 9: Negative cycles
- DVD player or laptop
- Clips related to 'Strange Situation' (Mary Ainsworth), 'Still Face' (Edward Tronick), etc.
- Homework sheet: Theme 2

FOCUS

- Importance of attachment and social-emotional development as a foundation for child development
- Babies' and children's communications

The main focus of this theme is the development of a child's attachment to their parental figure. This includes conversations on attachment in more detail and introduces the theme of stress and emotional regulation in babies, young children and adults.

Where possible, the parent(s) discuss this theme in a one to one session without their child.

KEY MESSAGES

- Babies and young children have strong, difficult feelings to manage that affect them both physically and emotionally - being hurt, frightened, hungry, tired, upset, lonely, jealous, angry, left out, etc. The baby or young child signals these needs to adults with attachment behaviours like calling, crying, clinging and staying close to the adult. Alongside this you can think of the parent's emotional response to the child's signals that help them to grow and thrive, being mindful of how the parent's feelings affect their responsiveness to their child too.
- These discussions can be wide-ranging, depending on the particular issues affecting the parent-child relationship. Clinical judgement is needed in terms of timing for these discussions and may include some of the following.
  - When the child is signalling needs they may be also experiencing stress, or even a sense of threat to their well-being; and this may be perceived or real on the baby's part. (This addresses some parents' dismissal of their baby experiencing fear/threat.) This theme may need to be approached differently for parents who have immediate safeguarding risks to themselves and their child, depending on whether they are able to acknowledge the risks.
  - Acknowledge that some children have developed ways of managing stress/worries by looking like they don't care, but who then attempt to self-regulate by being passive, very active or over-excited.
  - Acknowledge the immediate risk faced by some parents; their experience that neither they nor their child is safe from danger.

Conversely, for some parents who are not in touch with the risks, it can be helpful to start with everyday examples of how unpredictable situations or experiences can cause upset and stress for a child, especially if observed by the therapist.
  - Recognise that when babies and young children communicate to adults, they want their parents' support, care and love, that there is a demand on a parent's time and energy. Alongside this are the positive consequences for the child of developing confidence and security.

- A discussion on attachment can be introduced with general statements about the different ways babies and young children communicate their emotional needs, including those more vulnerable emotions/states when upset, hurt or scared. Some illustrations of how a child can struggle to communicate their needs may be helpful and relevant. Again clinical judgement is needed in selecting the most helpful resources for a parent that illustrate different patterns of attachment scenarios, i.e. when the child is stressed through a separation from a parent showing when the attachment system should 'kick in'. Online video clips of parents and children create the opportunity to discuss but not attribute blame. They can be useful as a way to think about how to build on what is working well and make changes that could help further.

- According to the specific presentation of the parent–child relationship and the insight of the parent at this point in time, one or more of the following can be used.
  - **Example of a secure attachment:** the therapist can create a brief narrative for the video and hear the parent's response. Key points relate to: how the child expresses emotion and signals their needs; that the parent responds to these with support; how the child quickly recovers emotionally as they get the comfort they need from the parent and returns to playing. Talk about the importance of this on an emotional level as well as the child being ready to engage with play and 'learning' sooner.
  - **Example of an avoidant attachment:** again this involves creating a brief narrative and hearing the parent's response. Key points relate to: how the child is not showing that they miss the parent; the child may give subtle and mixed responses to their parent, e.g. turning/looking away; they have no approach for showing their feelings and needs; more mechanical and limited play. Discuss the evidence that the child is not managing as they are known to be more

stressed (with raised and prolonged cortisol compared to a secure child) and how this affects their ongoing play and engagement/development. Composite examples can be helpful to show that the child's signals as well as the parent's responses are seen as key contributors to the relationship and interaction.

  - **Example of an ambivalent/resistant attachment:** the therapist can create a brief narrative and hear the parent's response. Key points relate to: how the child moves between demanding contact with the parent, then rejecting the parent's input; child often fussing and unable to settle with any play or the parent; how after the separation the child cannot make use of the comfort or attention of the adult to calm down and interact in a social way nor return to play. It may be helpful to recognise times when there is ordinary resistance, e.g. a child who is frustrated because they are not allowed to get something and who pulls away when the parent is trying to calm them, making the distinction between occasional behavioural issues and more entrenched patterns. Again composite examples can help to widen the discussion and may trigger links to the parent's and child's experience.

- Thinking with birth parents about change: through the intervention, parents and children are finding new ways to be together, talk and play, and this can take time to feel comfortable. Acknowledge that past experiences shape how individuals develop ways to cope with the pressures at any particular time. Also acknowledge how these strategies may not work as well when a context changes and how a child or adult can continue to use their way of interacting and communicating with others, e.g. a child continues to be self-reliant and 'rejecting' towards a parent who is trying to connect in different ways with their child.

- Thinking with adoptive parents or foster carers about change: acknowledge the process of change as per the discussion with birth parents above, but perhaps expand on the impact of past experiences on the current behaviours and responses of the baby/child. Reflect together on how this in turn can impact on their efforts to care for a child when they have not had that shared history. Acknowledge the entrenched nature of some behaviours, however subtle these may be, and how even when positive change is seen, the 'old' behaviours/interactions may resurface when the child is under greater stress, e.g. at a time of transition, or change in scheduled contact with birth parents.

- Thinking about the reciprocal nature of relationships: **Handout 5: To and fro of the parent–child relationship** can be useful as a visual depiction of this theme, and as a tool to talk about how the cycles of interaction impact on both parent and child. The timing of and extent of these discussions is linked to the individual family's needs and presentation, and may be addressed later in the intervention. A general discussion or use of **Handout 8: Positive cycles** and **Handout 9: Negative cycles** with non-specific examples of how people respond to one another helps to normalise this dynamic in all relationships. You can then decide whether to introduce more specific issues for that parent and child (e.g. repeating experiences from their own childhood, responding 'in kind' to the child) as the discussion progresses, bearing in mind the level of engagement in the therapeutic work.

TRANSITION TO NEXT SESSION/HOMEWORK

This will be included on an individual basis. All the homework sheets are designed to be used as a prompt for parents or can be filled in briefly and simply with images rather than much writing.

If it seems helpful, the parent can take away **Homework sheet: Theme 2** (where the parent is an observer of emotional states and responses in the child).

The sheet asks the parent to refer to a time and emotional state that they saw their child experiencing and then mark how they felt in the parental section on feelings.

Theme 3

Caring for your child – the ups and downs

RESOURCES

- Range of play materials and books for child's developmental level/interests
- Handouts:
  - Handout 8: Positive cycles
  - Handout 9: Negative cycles
  - Handout 10: Development of emotional regulation in children
- Homework sheet: Theme 3

FOCUS

- Practical play session
- Engaging with parent to observe and notice child's actions
- Feedback and discussion with parent about child's signals and feelings
- Parent's feelings and responses

This is the first practical play session starting the 'live' parent and child relationship work. The approaches to support this theme are detailed in Chapter 5, under the heading of 'Initial sessions' on page 95.

Theme 3 introduces the joint approach of the therapist and parent noticing what the child is doing and beginning to find a shared language and understanding of how the child responds in the 'here and now'. Alongside this there can be reflection with the parent about their responses and feelings.

Thought is given to the type of play materials that the parent and child feel more confident with, being mindful of the interests of the child and the parent from the assessment sessions.

KEY MESSAGES

- Take some time to address the fact that this is a new situation for the parent and child, even if they are in a familiar environment like the family home, and more so if the intervention is delivered somewhere new (e.g. a Children's Centre or Health Clinic). Acknowledge the presence of the therapist and the fact that they are still a relative stranger to the child. If in the family home, recognise that this is their environment and discuss/agree how/where the work will take place; the therapist can introduce suggestions and negotiate at an appropriate pace.
- The type of activity and interaction opportunities will vary greatly according to the age of the child and the specific presentation of the child and parent-child relationship. However, a common theme in this session is establishing a focus with the parent on the child's responses and interactions, and containing the parent when they are being closer with their child. The play is generally unstructured but the therapist can suggest more scaffolding to support both the parent and child.
- Revisit with the parent and child the role that the therapist will take. This will have been talked about in the feedback or an introductory session but it can be helpful to reiterate that the parent-child relationship is being prioritised. The therapist will not actively engage the child but

orientate them to the parent in general. If appropriate, give messages to the child so that they hear your intention to support the importance of their relationship with the parent.

- Along with the engagement of the parent, the main focus is to articulate micro-interactions as they occur between parent and child. Note the positive ones, beginning to reflect on what helps to maintain them as well as what can make it hard to do so. Some examples may include the following.
  - Therapist makes observations about interactions, however fleeting, noting the parent and child's response.
  - Where the child expresses a need, or where there is an absence of a communication of need, the therapist may articulate this and see/hear the parent's response. Use a stepped approach to suggest small ways that the parent might reach out, if appropriate to that moment, e.g. if a child resists being close, the parent could put a hand on the child's back to comfort them, or when the child hurts themselves but doesn't cry, help the parent to acknowledge the hurt, even if providing physical comfort may be too hard for the parent and child.
  - The therapist may offer observations and thoughts about the child's behaviour and responses, e.g. a child turning away to self-regulate, a baby's signals of anticipation of a response from their parent, a child's readiness to engage, their interest (however brief) in their parent, a child who is hard to comfort, a child clinging to their parent but who is angry.
  - Examples of more challenging interactions can be gently explored. As situations arise in the play and interaction, questions can be asked such as: 'Is this one of the times when you feel like they don't want you/want you to be involved?' Clinical judgement is needed here as it may be helpful to let the interaction run and prompt the adult to try a new way of relating. Or it may be helpful for a parent just to persevere with a communication with the child rather than explore their feelings at this point.
  - Think about the child's communications, e.g. a child may continue to reject/resist when the parent's response is positive, leaving the parent feeling they are not getting it 'right'. Acknowledge their efforts to connect as being helpful and that the baby/child has got a bit 'stuck'. Also acknowledge that it is hard to keep trying when the baby does not respond immediately and how it can take time for the baby to respond differently.

- A homework review from the last session can take place where appropriate. This could include picking up on the parent's feelings in their examples where they felt positive (joy, pride) or negative feelings (hurt, helpless) in response to their child's interactions/signals to them. If appropriate, explore how it made them respond in turn. Where applicable, acknowledge the positive attempts they made to reach out to their child.

TRANSITION TO NEXT SESSION/HOMEWORK

This will be included on an individual basis.

Homework sheet: Theme 3 focuses on moments when the parent recognises when their child may be more difficult to care for and what feelings were evoked in them. They are asked to note their feelings and then to try and think what their child may be feeling.

Theme 4

Tuning into your child's likes, dislikes and feelings

RESOURCES

- Range of play activities/toys/books.
- Handouts:
  - Handout 10: Development of emotional regulation in children
  - Handout 11: Running commentary: babies
  - Handout 12: Running commentary: toddler+
  - Handout 13: Parenting stress
- Homework sheet: Theme 4

FOCUS

- Practical play session
- Feedback and discussion with the parent about their child's signals or feelings
- Parent's feelings and responses
- Following the child's lead

The main focus of this session is on how to develop a child's curiosity and exploration. The parent is helped to understand and communicate their understanding of the child's interests and to follow their child's attention and interests.

This includes conversations with the parent to think about their child's own feelings, thoughts, likes/dislikes; that the child has a mind of their own. You can also make the link between this and greater self-confidence and emotional resilience for their child when they face challenges in the future.

KEY MESSAGES

- The child is taking some control and leading the play to some degree, and the match with their developmental stage and past experience is considered. The child's style of play and how they involve others will be known from assessment, e.g. being self-reliant or demanding of others' attention.
- Keep in mind that the child having 'control' can be difficult for some parents who may feel anxious or uncomfortable about feeling 'controlled' by their child. (This may be especially relevant where parents have experienced past abusive or coercive relationships.) As the child takes some control, and a parent follows the child's lead, the therapist supports and pays attention to the parent's responses and feelings.
- Acknowledge the different roles that parents have to negotiate; sometimes having a nurturing role towards their child, and other times allowing the child to take a lead and be more separate and independent. Having an open discussion about this helps to normalise the different feelings this may evoke for parents.
- There is a balance between the child having enough control to explore and having a feeling of mastery, along with the parent providing scaffolding and emotional regulation when needed. This avoids the child becoming overwhelmed. When this balance is 'right', the child can feel safe to develop and learn.
- Talk about how the parent helps to provide the scaffolding for their child to explore and learn through play. Explore the idea that it doesn't have to be 'all or nothing'. It's important to discuss this, especially if the parent feels rejected by the child's wish to be more autonomous or becomes anxious/controlling when the child takes charge.
- Discuss the child's feelings and wishes as they play and find a language with the parent to describe these so they can be named in a way that feels right to them. Acknowledge that both the positive and negative feelings of the child may need regulation as they can all be hard for the child to manage. Alongside this there should be an acknowledgment of the parent's feelings.

- Use the ideas in **Handout 11: Running commentary: babies** or **Handout 12: Running commentary: toddler+** in the session – where the parent makes simple comments on what they see their child doing or being interested in. You can talk about their use in everyday life at home too when the child does ordinary activities like washing their hands or eating. These are opportunities for the parent to be thoughtful as they talk about the child's wishes, preferences and feelings.
- There is the opportunity to video some of the play in the session if the parent is comfortable with this and has given written consent.
- The therapist supports the interaction and play with both parent and child, helping to extend the communication between them, using the 'parent–child live' techniques described in Chapter 5.
- The amount of time the parent and child will engage in joint, focused play will vary; the therapist can then give time to the parent to reflect together on how they experienced this and their thoughts on their child's experience.

TRANSITION TO NEXT SESSION/HOMEWORK
This will be included on an individual basis.

Homework sheet: Theme 4 asks the parent to note a moment at home when they read or played together, recording what they did and how it went, using the star system on the sheet.

Theme 5

Having choices and knowing when to say 'no'

RESOURCES
- Range of play activities/toys/books.
- Handouts:
  - Handout 14: Attachment and limit setting and Setting boundaries
- List of parent–child play activities for parent
- Homework sheet: Theme 5

FOCUS
- Introducing new/varied types of play and communication
- Noticing child's states and cues for engagement and 'breaks'
- Attachment and 'limit setting'

This session follows on from the previous theme in looking at how the parent can feel more confident in allowing their child to take the lead in play and social interaction, as well as allowing them to make appropriate choices in everyday life.

It keeps in mind the idea of reciprocity – the 'to and fro' of the relationship – and how this interpersonal experience is the foundation of the child's emotional well-being and stability. It also raises the issue of when a parent needs to set some limits around the child, linking in with emotional recognition and regulation.

KEY MESSAGES

- The session may continue with a similar type of play that the parent and child feel comfortable with or it may introduce more unstructured, symbolic or messy play (this will involve discussion beforehand with the parent). This session can be graded to be more or less challenging to the parent as you support them to follow the child in play that may raise emotive issues for both, e.g. doll figures that enact upsetting or aggressive behaviour in a play narrative.
- It is helpful to discuss ideas relating to how babies and children 'up-regulate' and 'down-regulate' as this gives more understanding about the child's underlying emotional state and describes the reason for the child taking 'breaks' from interaction. These can be noted and articulated as they arise in the 'live' work.
- The theme of attachment and limit setting may be introduced for parents and toddlers; this is not as relevant to parents with very young babies. (A discussion with parents of babies can be useful in order to hear the parent's view on discipline and gain an understanding of their personal scripts regarding this.)
- Acknowledge the challenge of setting reasonable limits on the child's demands while remaining available to give the child emotional support when they are frustrated or overwhelmed. Providing support/love with limit-setting is hard!
- Practical fictional examples can be helpful to look at with parents which then can lead to them thinking of their own more emotive experiences. These create an opportunity to explore the relational aspects, e.g. that it is difficult to work out if the child is trying to control or whether they use asking for food to communicate that they need comfort. Consider

how signals can become muddled and the child may only be seen as 'controlling'.

- Flag and discuss the importance of both the emotional and behavioural sides to these interactions and the need for the child to have support and regulation from the parent.
- An integral message is that if children are allowed some autonomy and choice they are less likely to 'battle' with the parent when the adult does have to take charge.
- Focus on the moments of shared enjoyment, highlighting strengths. Where parents remain quite controlling of the child it is helpful to acknowledge their good intentions. Equally there will be containment for the parent by reflecting on the difficult moments and, if appropriate, their anxiety or anger.

TRANSITION TO NEXT SESSION/HOMEWORK

This will be included on an individual basis. **Homework sheet: Theme 5** sets a goal for the parent to try a couple of activities from the session or the activities list at home, and to allow the child some choices in how the play develops.

You can also encourage the parent to let the child make some choice each day – with toys, food, clothes – if this seems appropriate and realistic at this stage.

THEME 6

Responding to your child's signals and communications

RESOURCES

- Video clips of parent–child interactions (from YouTube or published DVDs)
- Handouts:
  - Handout 8: Positive cycles
  - Handout 9: Negative cycles
  - Handout 10: Development of emotional regulation in children
  - Handout 15: How babies interact and regulate emotions
- Homework sheet: Theme 6

FOCUS

- Introducing new/varied types of play and communication
- Noticing child's states and cues for engagement and 'breaks'
- Attachment and limit setting

This session focuses on the idea that children need varying attention and proximity from their parent from one moment to another. This extends ideas already touched on that babies and children use engaging and disengaging as part of a normal way to help regulate their emotions and physical/body systems. The 'Still Face' study video clips or general parent–child video interactions may be helpful to show examples of how babies down-regulate in order to manage strong emotions and physical tension.

This session can also introduce the concept of the child being afraid of objects or people around them and that adults may unintentionally play a part in this.

KEY MESSAGES

- Have a general discussion about everyone, including children, having their own personal space and thresholds for noise, stimulation and activity. If helpful, talk about the ideas from the Brazelton assessment for neonates which demonstrates how babies are born with preferences from birth for more or less stimulation, different types of sensory input, and temperature.

- You could also reflect with the parent on examples from their own experience if this seems clinically appropriate and in tune with their capacity for self-reflection. For example, the parent thinks of a memory where they may have felt overwhelmed and needed to withdraw, or conversely had become more active, or a time when excitement was mixed with fear.

- Some children will have adapted to stress by using self-regulatory strategies as a standard response to feeling dysregulated; how an individual child responds can be discussed, e.g. looking away, self-soothing or using constant motion. This conversation may be more possible earlier in the work if the child is with a new caregiver (foster/adoptive parent). This may also be possible with birth parents if the stress the family has been under is already acknowledged, and the link has been made about how the child (and parent) needed to adapt to their previous experiences.

- The concept of behaviours being adaptive at the time of stress/trauma but then becoming used automatically as the 'norm' can be discussed. The impact of this on the parent and child will be different and needs reflecting on sensitively. For example, the parent may have recovered from a mental health condition but finds that their child does not then respond differently to them, creating upset and guilt in the parent. The work supports the parent to help the child in turn to give up these behaviours; the notion of 'past their sell-by date'.
- The notion that a child can be afraid of objects or people around them can be introduced and that adults may unintentionally play a part in this. This concept is explored more in later sessions but can be referred to here as a starting point.
- In the play activity the parent can be supported to notice the child's signals and communicate these to them. This helps the child to feel others understand their point of view and that they are being taken seriously.
- It is important to understand the parent's view of 'stimulation' for their child; some parents may unintentionally be intrusive through anxiety or in an effort to get a response, while others may think it is better to leave a child to learn on their own.
- Hypothetical examples of children being overwhelmed by stimulation, e.g. prolonged tickling, could be discussed.
- A child's signals that communicate they want more or less input from the adult can be thought about. Use examples from their child where possible.
  - Signals that the child wants more involvement can include babbling, calling, looking, smiling or crying.
  - Signals that the child wants more space can include looking down or to the side, turning their head or body away, ceasing to play, self-soothing or becoming restless.
- **Handout 8: Positive cycles** and **Handout 9: Negative cycles** can be used to explore the patterns of interaction in relation to the child's needs/signals and the parent's feelings and responses, e.g. understanding the child needing space, feeling rejected or not needed, responding 'in kind' to the child.

TRANSITION TO NEXT SESSION/HOMEWORK

This will be included on an individual basis.

Homework sheet: Theme 6 provides cues for the parent to look for and to note the signals in their child about needing to regulate. There is space for the parent to note what they did and how the child responded.

Theme 7

Understanding your child's emotions

RESOURCES

- Handouts:
  - Handout 16: Emotions
  - Handout 17: Mixed emotions
- Children's books on feelings; resources, e.g. 'feelings faces'
- DVDs on children's emotions or YouTube, e.g. 'Growing an emotional brain'

FOCUS

- Play-based session
- Exploring the child's emotions
- Articulating and naming feelings with the child

This session's focus is on recognising emotional responses and states in young babies and children and exploring how they (and adults) can be aware of and express strong emotions.

The theme also introduces the idea of children experiencing mixed emotions about one experience or event.

KEY MESSAGES

- Previous sessions' themes have focused on the parent tuning into their child's intentions and underlying emotional states. This is now extended to explore the parent's views on those emotional states their child experiences and which are, in the parent's view, acceptable to express. The handouts/videos are a useful starting point to think about their beliefs and 'scripts' relating to specific emotions. This is particularly relevant to strong emotions that may now, or in the past, have been described as 'unacceptable' or have felt unmanageable, e.g. jealousy, anger, fear.

- There are many ways that this key topic can be explored and so the ideas below are suggestions for possible avenues that have been taken when talking with parents. The order is not set out to suggest any priority as this is individual to each family.
  - It is important to understand the parent's 'scripts' from childhood. It is also helpful to think back with them to times when they were young (if the parent can engage with this). It allows more exploration of which strong feelings they can recall being recognised and accepted, or not, and how others responded to them at the time, e.g. receiving support, or being dismissed or ignored.
  - **Handout 16: Emotions** can help facilitate a discussion as it is visual and gives time to the parent to consider a wide range of feelings. (They can circle those that they felt as a child and/or as an adult and which are uncomfortable or 'unacceptable' in their mind.)
  - Encourage the parent to think about these and other emotions in their child. and reflect on how they recognise and respond to them. Use examples from the parent-child work and previous discussions to link it with their everyday experiences.
  - **Handout 17: Mixed emotions** is one way of exploring how feelings can be confusing, with one feeling masking another at times, e.g. sadness underlying anger, or excitement covering fear. Think about specific examples of this for them or their child and help the parent to recognise when their child had mixed feelings and felt torn or confused by an experience.
  - Use creative activities to explore this with the child and parent, e.g. books with narratives or poems about different emotions, or drawing emotions on a simple body map, or making 'feeling faces' using paper plates.
  - Use video clips from their own videos (if these are available and the parent agrees) to review moments when different emotions were expressed between them and their child.

- For some parents it is helpful to think about how children with social-emotional development delays or difficulties need more help than the average child to manage their emotions. This relates to issues of adversity, trauma, illness or other stressors that the child and family have faced.

- The progress of a child's emotional development may be at odds with other aspects of their functioning and may need unpicking with the parent to see that more emotional support/regulation is needed. For example, the child may have advanced speech or cognitive ability but may be easily distressed or vulnerable to changes or frustrations.
- Reflect on the difference between accepting and recognising feelings in a child, to accepting behaviours in the child. Difficult or inappropriate behaviour must be managed but the underlying feelings need to be reflected on. Discuss this being one of the ways that a child's behaviour itself can be regulated.

TRANSITION TO NEXT SESSION/HOMEWORK

This will be included on an individual basis.

Handout 16: Emotions and **Handout 17: Mixed emotions** can be given to the parent to use when thinking of a situation in the week. They can circle all the emotions that apply in a chosen moment in themselves and the child.

Theme 8

Feeling scared – when our 'buttons get pressed'

RESOURCES

- Handouts:
  - Handout 1: Commonly held beliefs about babies and children
  - Handout 13: Parenting stress
  - Handout: 18: How buttons get pressed
- Video clips from DVDs or YouTube illustrating anxiety responses, e.g. Still Face
- Homework sheet: Theme 8a
- Homework sheet: Theme 8b

FOCUS

- Recognising anxiety/fear in the child and in the parent
- Parenting stress
- Triggers for parent and child
- Responding to the child in the 'here and now'

The timing of this theme is important as it brings strong and often unprocessed emotions to the fore. It is often explored over more than one session with the handouts/resources, but is intrinsic to much of the intervention.

It introduces the idea that there are times when the child or baby is frightened – this can be in general situations and possibly at times when they are frightened by the parent. It helps the parent to recognise that there are experiences that the child may be fearful of or stressed by, but that adults may not see as such. The conversations will also focus on the parent's recognition of anxiety in themselves, and the triggers that cause it, including specific ones from their child. At the same time, it is important to be mindful of the history of stress, loss and/or trauma that they have experienced.

The theme moves on to thinking about ways in which the parent can be more aware of when anxiety and fear are evoked in themselves and their child, and how they can contain these feelings so they impact less on the relationship between them and their child.

KEY MESSAGES

- It may be helpful to begin with ordinary examples of how a child may experience threat or fear that are not easy for the parent to recognise. This may be particularly relevant for babies who are more avoidant and show little emotion themselves, or when the child demonstrates their stress by active/disorganised behaviour which can then be seen as 'difficult' or 'bad'.
- The therapist will have in mind issues relating to the parent's past experience of receiving support, or not, for anxieties/fears. They can gently introduce links between these and their current beliefs/coping mechanisms, e.g. by using **Handout 1: Commonly held beliefs about babies and children** and examples of triggers arising from the live parent–child work (the child taking more control in play eliciting worry in the parent).
- Create space to reflect that a parent's difficulty in recognising fear or anxiety may link to their child having defences that inhibit them showing these emotions directly and/or that the parent is out of touch with these feelings in themselves. (This may arise from traumatic, neglectful childhood experience, insecure attachments, adult relationships involving abuse/trauma, etc.) Recognition of the stress evoked in parents and their feelings needs to be addressed sensitively and at an appropriate pace.

- In the first instance, the notion that an adult can be the source of fear and anxiety for a child can be introduced by using fictional examples, e.g. an adult being playful but frightening a child by jumping out from a hiding place. Some parents' personal thresholds for fear may be high as they have experienced an overwhelming amount themselves when younger, and so they can in turn dismiss incidents for their child as insignificant. For some, the idea that a parent is a protector and comforter to their child may be strange or feel alien to them.
- Acknowledge that it is confusing and alarming for both adults and children if the person they feel close to is the same person who is frightening them. Children and adults can feel stuck, paralysed and overwhelmed. The therapist keeps in mind the developmental consequences for a child who is frightened too often and how this undermines their capacity to think, interact, concentrate and learn. Smaller specific examples can be thought about with the parent to illustrate the impact on their child; these should be conveyed with empathy for the adult's emotional experience too.
- Explore what scripts may come automatically to mind when the parent is triggered by their child. Some examples include: a parent immediately thinking 'he's making me ill'; a parent who was not believed about their own trauma as a child is provoked by their child not acting in the way they describe them to be; a misattribution is made to the child showing the parent up as 'a liar'.
- Where appropriate or possible, have a conversation about how the parent, if feeling threatened themselves, may 'respond in kind' and frighten their child in turn. This can be approached in different ways depending on the relationship with the parent but it must be conveyed with empathy and be containing to the parent.
- **Handout 18: How buttons get pressed** helps to normalise that 'buttons get pressed' for all parents. It facilitates more discussion about the parent's own experience (or use of other online resources relating to parenting or trauma). This also helps to recognise the particular issues that upset or anger the parent and then in turn interfere with the relationship here and now with their child. Examples could include: baby/child crying or being demanding and needing a lot of attention; baby turning away and being more independent; child refusing the help or comfort offered by the parent.

- The 'live' work, as well as further reflective discussion with the parent, can focus on bringing this awareness to everyday activities; how quickly interactions can change from going smoothly to becoming 'disturbed' or difficult. It is important for the parent to recognise the strength of feelings evoked in them (and possibly the child) along with reflection on how this can be out of proportion to the actual events because of 'buttons' being pressed.
- Getting a measure of the number, type and strength of the triggers for the parent is important, recognising these emerge over time too. As mentioned, they vary greatly for each person, and may be an indication of the need for further support in terms of individual therapy for the parent.

TRANSITION TO NEXT SESSION/HOMEWORK

This is included on an individual basis as before, and is particularly important to consider here as this is such an emotive theme. For many parents the discussions will take place within sessions only.

Homework sheet: Theme 8a asks the parent what buttons get pressed with their child and what feelings are evoked in them, with any 'scripts' that come to mind at the time.

Homework sheet: Theme 8b includes a section for 'How did you respond?'. If the parent wishes to approach this between sessions, it may be helpful to arrange a phone call to support them in the week.

Theme 9

Caring for children when 'buttons get pressed'

RESOURCES

- Prepared materials for the parent-child play task.
- Handout:
  - Handout 13: Parenting stress
- Homework sheet: Theme 9

FOCUS

- Recognising anxiety/fear/anger in the child and parent
- Parenting stress
- Triggers for the parent and child
- Responding to the child in the 'here and now'

This theme and Theme 8 are interlinked, with the ideas and approaches being used flexibly in response to the clinical context. Theme 8 addressed the ideas around the recognition of fear/anxieties in the parent and child. Theme 9 focuses on how the parent can regulate feelings in themselves and those in their child. This can help them to try to disentangle the feelings and prevent them from impacting negatively on patterns of interaction and the parent-child relationship.

KEY MESSAGES

- Within the remit of this intervention you can help parents to become more aware of their own individual responses, and support them by normalising the notion that a dynamic operates between past and present, raising strong emotions in response to their child's cues or behaviours. It can reassure parents that they are not 'failing' or being 'weak'; the reverse is true as they will become more confident in managing the feelings that arise naturally and will feel a greater sense of control and ease.

- Discussions consider how the parent manages the feelings in the moment when they are with their child and how this can impact positively on their relationship and day-to-day experiences. For example, if a parent becomes aware that their anxiety about their child not eating is linked to reasons from their own childhood, they can reflect on this, which can help to contain their worry. In turn, this will help them to not pass on pressure to the child. This is important because conflict or tension around meals can lead to the child eating even less, creating a vicious circle.

- It is helpful to return to thinking about the child's individual capacity for emotional and self-regulation, as this can vary so much. It is an important piece of the relational puzzle and gives the parent insight into what support their child may need, reflecting the two-way nature of how emotions from the parent and child impact on one another. Although the responsibility to instigate change remains largely with the parent, recognition of the child's contribution is important for the parent.
- **Handout 13: Parenting stress** or other similar resources can support parents to think of ways they can manage their own angry or upset feelings at 'trigger' points. This is then followed up within the live work to support them putting these strategies into practice.
- This could be a time in the intervention to agree with the parent the inclusion of play activities that may be harder for them to negotiate and manage, recognising that this could be a time when 'buttons are pressed' for the parent and/or child, e.g. sensory messy play, or symbolic play with aggressive themes.
- Another option is to focus on an everyday task in a session, e.g. feeding, if the parent has highlighted this as a difficulty. A further option is to discuss with the parent tackling a specific behaviour or dynamic with their child that feels 'stuck' and emotive, e.g. the parent being able to talk with another adult while their child is present or transition points at the start/end of sessions.
- The techniques in Chapter 5 are used to facilitate both the live work between the parent and child and the follow-up reflective discussion with the parents.

TRANSITION TO NEXT SESSION/HOMEWORK

This is included on an individual basis as before, and is particularly important to consider here as this is such an emotive theme. For many parents the discussions will take place within sessions only.

Homework sheet: Theme 9 follows on from Theme 8 specifically. It includes a section on 'What did you do?'. If the parent wishes to look at this between sessions, it may be helpful to arrange a phone call to support them in the week.

Theme 10

Playing together

RESOURCES

- Individual Activity templates
- Homework sheet: Theme 10

FOCUS

- Play-based sessions
- Exploring changes and closeness in the relationship between parent and child
- Articulating and naming feelings for the child and parent

In the latter part of the intervention it is useful to have a more specific focus on the progress of the child's development and the relationship. Think whether there are any other ways to introduce joint play that is positive and enjoyable.

The therapist supports the parent to come up with suggestions and, if it is helpful for the parent, they can be tried out within sessions or in everyday life to strengthen their confidence in their knowledge and intuition about their child.

KEY MESSAGES

- The new activity/play will be chosen with the aim of extending more curious and explorative play together with the parent. The different dynamic this brings to the relationship needs consideration. For example, the play could introduce more close physical contact, higher levels of excitement or conversely more relaxing, quiet moments between them.
- Recognise that new ways of relating, especially if creating moments of greater intimacy and shared emotion, will need support and some reflection on the feelings and responses evoked.
- The therapist may have a role in helping to grade new activities alongside the parent so that the demands on the child and parent for proximity, eye contact and physical closeness are considered.
- Return to ideas around emotional and physical regulation of the child and supporting the parent to respond to this, while acknowledging their feelings in the moment. Give positive feedback to the parent to

persevere with new approaches and give affirmation of how they are creating essential foundations for their child's future potential. This discussion can be tailored to the individual aspects of their child's development.

- Discuss what feels comfortable for the parent, and child, and think together about how the child is communicating their feelings and preferences for the new kinds of contact with their parent. Acknowledge it can take some time and repetition for new ways of relating and being together to feel more normal.

TRANSITION TO NEXT SESSION/HOMEWORK

This is included on an individual basis, as before.

The parent can add a list of possible activities to **Homework sheet: Theme 10** that they would like to try at home, with the option to then rate them.

Theme 11

Transitions/saying goodbye

RESOURCES

- Play materials

FOCUS

- Reflections on the intervention process
- Progress made in the child and the parent–child relationship
- Acknowledging feelings around ending
- Making use of resources, including signposting
- Setting a time for review (if this is due to take place)

The theme of transitions will have been addressed frequently within the clinical sessions and around therapy breaks during the intervention.

The focus here mainly addresses the ending of the intervention sessions and considers how this can be approached with the child, parent and their network.

A previously agreed activity may be chosen and prepared as a way of marking the last session.

KEY MESSAGES

- Have a discussion with the parent and child about their experience of the intervention. This gives an opportunity to reflect on the important moments and issues for them, and the progress and changes they have made. Depending on the age of the child, they may have quite clear memories or thoughts that they can articulate and this can be powerful for the parent to hear.
- There is a chance to think about the parent's strengths and skills and to reinforce their capacity to be in tune with their child, using their awareness of their child's needs.
- Acknowledge and discuss the feelings that are evoked by the ending for both the adult and the child (although this is often raised across more than one session as the intervention nears its conclusion). This can often include sadness and anxieties about coping but can also be a time to feel hope and pride in what they have achieved.
- If video has been used in the assessment and/or intervention, copies of these are made and made available for the family. Still photos from the video that captured some of the positive moments between the parent and their child can also be made and given.
- Discuss and signpost local resources, including other community services or organisations. This supports the family to continue to build their own network.
- Where there is a system in place for a review assessment to be carried out, arrangements for this can be made. This can have a 'holding' effect for the family.

7 Supervision and case review

Clinical supervision is essential for all professionals involved in this work. Ideally this would be with other professionals who are familiar with the SUSI model. Due to the emotional engagement that is essential for the therapist's work to be successful, a more 'hands off' objective view of the process helps the therapist not to become too enmeshed.

Providing a space to review and reflect on the relationship between the therapist and child and/or parent leads to good, effective practice. This remains true, irrespective of the practitioners' experience and training. It also supports fidelity to the SUSI therapeutic modality, allowing for the application and adaptation of this within appropriate boundaries in order to meet the individual needs of the client.

The need for ongoing supervision during implementation

Overall a significant level of supervision is required for staff undertaking the SUSI assessments, interventions and liaison work with other professionals and the wider network. There are several reasons for this in both the SUSI study and in our clinical service which may also apply to other settings, for example the majority of staff:

- may be relatively inexperienced in the field of clinical work with babies and young children
- are undertaking additional training in a specific model of care
- may be introducing a new model in a multi-agency context.

There is evidence that for those practitioners undertaking further post-graduate training in evidence-based practice, they may not continue using the techniques learned in the immediate months post training. One of the most common reasons given for this is the lack of supervision and consultation available following the training. Kavanagh et al. (1993) found that, within a group of professionals who had been trained in a specific Adult Mental Health intervention, only a minority were using the techniques learned in the following three years.

In the field of early intervention with young children and parents, the difficulty in successfully implementing evidence-based interventions has been highlighted (NICE, 2012), with specific examples of workforce training not leading to changes in practice.

A framework for supervision and case reviews

The different elements of the SUSI model training programme are covered in greater detail in Chapter 9. Here we will focus on how individual case supervision and team-based case review meetings were organised for the project team, a framework which can be adapted to other contexts.

A supervision structure was created for formal, individual supervision and a weekly team clinical meeting was established for all therapists, with consideration given to the match between supervisor and supervisee.

Note that, when the model is being delivered in a clinical service or in a clinical research setting, the researchers or equivalent assistant psychology posts have the same supervision needs. Therefore, the term 'researchers' can be used interchangeably with other assistant practitioners according to the context of the work. In the SUSI study, the researchers were allocated an individual supervisor to discuss the direct work with the families. This was because they had a high level of contact with distressed people on a daily basis. Specific research supervision was provided on a regular basis for the researchers as a team, with a weekly meeting for consultation with the study's Research Consultant.

The timing and frequency of supervision for each member of the team was considered based on their previous CAMHS and other clinical experience, grade, professional and post-graduate training.

Individual supervision

In general, individual supervision was scheduled on a more frequent basis initially to:

- help support the therapist's integration into the team
- orientate them to new services and agencies' structures
- promote fidelity to the clinical model.

Following this period, there would be a minimum of monthly supervision, with the supervisor and supervisee establishing a contract for these meetings.

The clinical supervision meetings followed a standard process in which the supervisee and supervisor contributed to an agenda and then prioritised the identified tasks for the focus of their discussions. This focus varied across the stages of work in the assessment, intervention and review time-points for the families. It considered the engagement and direct work with families, as well as the liaison and collaboration with the network.

For example, when focusing on the initial assessment stage, the supervision discussion included detailed analysis of:

- individual assessments for a child and their family
- the infant/child's presentation
- the impact both from and contributing to the quality of relationship(s) with primary caregivers and other key figures.

In addition, the contribution of psychosocial, medical, cultural and environmental contextual factors were carefully considered. Significant care and thought were given to the writing up and formulation of the assessment (and subsequent reports). Therapists need support to be able to reflect on and communicate the material with both clarity as well as sensitivity.

Throughout these tasks, time was needed to reflect on the emotional impact on therapists of the direct contact with the child and family, and to consider how this added to our understanding of the clinical picture. Importantly, it also provided support to individual therapists who frequently experienced high levels of distress and trauma during visits and contacts with the families. As we know, these can engender strong emotional responses in professionals because they receive powerful and often unprocessed emotional communications from the children and adults. These include, among others, feelings of anxiety, frustration, anger and confusion, as well as the experience of being deskilled.

AREAS ROUTINELY COVERED IN INDIVIDUAL SUPERVISION

- Specific case information relating to referrals, recruitment and engagement was considered. Consideration was also given to concrete issues, e.g. timing of appointments, parent or child psychopathology or risk factors that may act as barriers to their participation.
- The assessment procedure had to be administered sensitively and the process was adapted to minimise anxiety for the family. For example, if a parent was very anxious, it could further heighten their stress to start with the questionnaires. Consideration as to how best to engage and build a therapeutic alliance with the parents and children in supervision was often needed.
- Reports were routinely discussed in individual supervision as it was vital that they were clear, brief and written in accessible language. They needed to clearly state the concerns while not being read as a criticism of the parents. The wording and tone of the reports was a delicate balance and staff needed time and support to communicate both complicated relationship dynamics and individual factors.
- Case notes were reviewed periodically to ensure that the assessment data and clinical work was accurately recorded to reflect the needs of individual cases. The clinical discussion gave the opportunity to think about the needs of each family and how best to tailor the SUSI model to meet these.
- Careful consideration of the assessment recommendations guided the feedback discussions and intervention planning with the family and the wider network. This helped address differing views in the wider network, and safeguarding thresholds where appropriate, regarding the child and family's well-being and functioning. Staff often required support to prepare for the feedback meetings so that the relevant issues could be raised and discussed in a constructive way.
- The emotional burden of the work on individual staff members was significant. While there were many positives as we witnessed the progress in children and parent's relationships, and emotional and developmental difficulties improved, staff also had to frequently hold considerable anxiety and uncertainty. Was this care 'good enough' for the child and within their timescales? Could parents be provided with sufficient care and input for their own needs? Staff are our main resource and both formal and informal supervision is needed to provide them with 'a secure base' of their own in the work setting.

- The delivery of the intervention was brought regularly to supervision to consider the child and family's response and progress, together with which techniques and intervention themes were helpful to use at different stages. New information or insights were often shared by the parent or observed by the therapist as the intervention proceeded. These informed next steps in the direct work and a decision as to how or when this might be shared with key workers in the wider network.
- Different agencies can hold very different views and impressions of parents (and children). Splits can occur, causing tensions between staff and services at times. However, these can be important communications about different aspects of the family and reflect parents' good intentions and strengths on the one hand and resistance, hostility and ambivalence on the other. Individual supervision helped the therapist understand these tensions while keeping a focus on the child's needs so a balanced representation and view could be communicated in multi-agency meetings.
- Decision-making forums with parents and the wider network took place according to need; post-assessment, during and after the intervention, as appropriate. Discussions about the frequency and purpose of these meetings in supervision helped to keep a focus on the child's progress, together with the awareness of other agencies' hopes about the impact of the intervention. It was important that the therapist was supported in order to be clear about their role and what might realistically be achieved. Again, supervision for the individual therapist ensured that the SUSI contribution remained focused on the child and parent to effect positive change in the child/parent relationship.

In addition to the scheduled supervision sessions, regular contact in between meetings was often required to address more urgent issues, e.g.:

- safeguarding concerns
- network liaison as new clinical information arose
- the submission of assessment and review reports to meet deadlines for cross-agency meetings.

As therapists were often highlighting areas of previously unidentified need, frequent support was required to help staff both engage families and deliver concise but complex information to the professional network.

Clinical case review team meetings

In a clinical service or project context, it is important to hold regular weekly team meetings for all therapists to attend. For the SUSI project, the meeting was led by a Team Lead and an agenda was drawn up at the start of each week, with the individual cases that therapists wished to bring for discussion.

Case discussion included different aspects of the work in order to:

- bring back more complex assessments
- review and reflect on the progress of an intervention
- consider specific inter-agency liaison and work
- review additional support and service involvement for specific needs of the child and/or adult highlighted during the intervention or reviews.

The case discussion included standard components such as:

- a brief history
- the assessment of the child's presenting issues, relationships and developmental profile
- the current family situation, including personal and environmental stressors
- the network context including statutory and legal context where applicable.

In addition, a detailed description and initial formulation of the parent-child interaction and relationship was presented, integrating information from the standardised measures and clinical observations. Insights from a description of the child's response to the therapists were described, together with the presentation of the adult's emotional/mental state.

The therapist identified the primary aim of bringing the case to the meeting and described what help they would like from the team. Key points and any decisions were recorded on a template for the allocated therapist, which could be reviewed in a future team meeting or individual supervision.

These meetings were valuable in terms of both supporting and extending the clinical work but also in sharing learning between therapists. The diversity of the populations and individual presentations resulted in a wide range of issues. The skill mix of the team, including experience of work within Adult Mental Health, with adolescents and Child Health settings, could be fully utilised in this forum.

In a setting where a team is being newly formed and therapists are implementing a new clinical model, the meetings can be used to revisit some of the specific clinical approaches and techniques to support learning and fidelity to the model.

8 Integration of work with other agencies

The work really helped us to make sense of how a child's experiences were presenting in their behaviour. It was also incredibly helpful in identifying what s/he most needed in the next stage of their life.

INDEPENDENT REVIEWING OFFICER

From a professional perspective, the assessment formulations were really helpful in gaining an understanding of the family and what we might build upon once the SUSI intervention was complete.

PARENTAL MENTAL HEALTH WORKER

We were able to do some joint visits with the SUSI worker when issues arose and this also helped improve the quality of support that the social workers provided to new families.

SOCIAL WORKER

Winnicott's statement that 'a baby alone doesn't exist' can be extended to individual families; they also do not exist on their own. Families that have a range of complex health, social and environmental needs require interventions to be firmly embedded in the community's multi-agency system.

Collaborative inter-agency work ensures better outcomes for the whole family. The families' involvement is vital as no matter how valid an intervention may be, it will not be effective if the family do not engage.

Darlington, Feeney and Rixon (2005) note that inter-agency collaboration is notoriously difficult to achieve. Effective collaboration is challenged by:

- the absence of basic information about available services
- poor knowledge of staff and skills available in other agencies
- a lack of systems culture
- lack of liaison.

Cleaver & Walker (2004) write about the importance of effective multi-agency working to deliver efficient and comprehensive services to families. An unappreciated advantage to integrated work is that families or wider family members may already be known to community agencies. Intergenerational problems are frequently known to the wider network and use of collective intelligence is important. Knowledge of what has and has not helped in the past can aid the approach to the family so that work can be delivered in as sensitive a way as possible.

High risk and vulnerable families

Services need to explore families' strengths so that, where possible, they can be supported and receive sufficient and targeted assistance to remain together, preventing further cycles of separation, abuse and neglect. The agency network also needs to have shared, articulated goals in order to review robustly the progress, or not, of the child's development and well-being. This informs next steps in a network care plan which requires strong collaboration and good working relationships with both the 'system' and the families.

This multi-agency collaboration needs to be not only at a strategic level but also at a grassroots level, particularly with 'high risk' families. This is so that proactive and preventative work can really happen. This facilitates the possibility of joint visits and joint assessments, and effective use of resources. For example, staff from agencies can:

- use each other's premises as appropriate
- agree aims of the work
- find effective ways of engaging the families.

SUSI therapists carried out assessments and interventions in Children's Centres, and met with parents in Children's Social Care (CSC) and Child Health buildings. This made sense to the staff and to the families so they had a real experience of the 'system' working together in order to clarify how best to respond to the range of identified needs. Research shows that better outcomes for children can be achieved through effective partnership work with families (Aldgate & Bradley, 1999; Cleaver, Unell & Aldgate, 2011).

Engagement of multi-agency stakeholders is fundamental to facilitate inter-agency practice and care planning. It is no easy task as even now services often struggle to agree a shared language and there continues to be different understandings of risk, mental illness, emotional well-being and the social-emotional developmental needs of children (Hetherington et al., 2002). However difficult this groundwork is to achieve, if the interfaces are not well negotiated, communication and service aims remain disjointed, with the possibility of service conflict and a poor service offered to children and families (Darlington, Feeney & Rixon, 2004).

The ability to accurately and sensitively identify which children and families need a service, and to respond quickly with the appropriate intervention or plan, is a challenge faced by all services working in this area. This has long been recognised in the work from the Audit Commission (1994) and Department of Health (DH 1995, 2000). Here the emphasis has been on a move away from work driven by risk and incidents, to work that encompasses a holistic approach to best identify the child's, and the family's, developmental and contextual needs and strengths. If individual circumstances and environmental factors are understood and considered, there is a better chance of success. For example, a family previously unknown to services presents in crisis after a bereavement of a close family member. If not attended to promptly, the strain on a family can lead to rapidly escalating difficulties and may necessitate statutory involvement.

Initiatives to implement a comprehensive multi-agency approach, such as the Assessment Framework (2000), have faced many challenges with services struggling under the demand and volume of work. In these pressured situations, staff have limited capacity to consider collaborative and systemic work (Darlington, Feeney & Rixon, 2005). In addition to the family crisis, complicated funding arrangements (Hudson, 2002) add pressure on services that already feel overburdened and present a challenge to multi-agency working (Scott, 2010).

Promoting integrated multi-agency work in SUSI

A collaborative multi-agency approach is often difficult to define and put into operation. However, it ensures open and respectful working together, where professional knowledge and skills are shared and differences of opinion and conflict can be thought about to reach a consensus for the family.

This collaborative approach was embedded as a consistent and articulated feature of the SUSI care pathway. In Chapter 2, the structure of the model is outlined, showing the formal and informal contact points with colleagues in partner agencies for communication and information sharing. For example, review meetings happened at specific time-points, e.g. the assessment feedback stage and intervention feedback. Depending on the needs of the child and family, or changes in the network, additional reviews were also arranged as necessary. Joint meetings were also scheduled with the families, when there were specific concerns and changes to the plan that needed consideration. Sometimes these meetings were scheduled because there was a change of social worker or other key professional, to ensure the momentum of the work was not lost and that the new members of staff had a good knowledge of the issues, as well as supporting the family with staff changes.

Throughout the SUSI work, other professionals or other family members were included as much as possible. For example, if in the initial phase a colleague (Health Visitor, nursery staff member, AMH worker) had an existing positive relationship with one of the parents, they would be invited to join the parents when we discussed their possible engagement. This gave the parents a greater opportunity to discuss any anxieties or questions they might have in relation to the work with a known, trusted person present, and the team could get to know the family's network better. When needed, this also helped to facilitate referral and access to other appropriate services for the parent or child.

CASE STUDY

A parent had a serious neurological condition that meant he found it hard to leave his home. His medical condition, although being treated, was impacting on his own mental health and at times he presented as paranoid, including in relation to his daughter. This was further compounded by his social isolation. Services were sympathetic to his condition and struggles as a parent. However, the reality was that he could not support his daughter to meet her developmental, social and emotional needs. The young toddler was frequently absent from nursery and remained at home with her frightened and anxious father. By providing clear evidence about the impact of this on the child, the network became aware of the urgency of the situation from the child's perspective and actively pursued additional resources for the father, including Adult Mental Health. It also helped the network develop a plan, so they could more accurately monitor the girl's development and emotional needs. ●●●

As described in earlier chapters, information and recommendations from the SUSI assessment and/or intervention could be challenging for both the families and the professionals, so they needed to be shared sensitively.

CASE STUDY

A care plan for a 3-year-old boy in foster care involved a permanent move to a family member on a Special Guardianship Order (SGO). During the introductions phase with the boy and the SG carer, it was clear that family members had minimised the impact on him when scheduled contact with his birth mother took place. This led to conflict in the network meetings as different aspects of the child's presentation were discussed and considered. The initial care plan for the SGO was challenged and caused frustration in the system. In order to get a helpful resolution and support the child, foster parent and staff, network meetings were held including senior staff and the plan was reconsidered in the light of the new information and in the best interests of the boy. ●●●

Burden of services on families

There is an obvious danger in multi-agency work: families might feel overburdened or confused about who they are seeing, what agencies they are from, and why each is involved. Indeed, this can be challenging for staff as several, and at times contrasting, views need to be taken into account.

If this work is well co-ordinated and follows common sense principles, then most problems can be avoided. Knowledge of other services and professional colleagues' roles helps to build a functioning network that can sensitively plan a reasonable schedule for the family. For example, if a parent and child were attending a Child Health or CSC appointment we could join the appointment if needed and/or request a room to use so the child and parent could be seen directly before or after by us. If the family was tired or stressed, it was possible to negotiate the length of the appointment. This had the added advantage of giving the family the message of a supportive, co-ordinated system around them. It was also clinically economic as information about the parent's/child's needs was shared and additional assessments accessed in a timely way, thus reducing stress for the family and therapists.

Awareness of partner agencies' timeframes

It is important to be aware of other professionals' timescales and pressures. While the model allows for flexibility in relation to appointment timing and venues for the parents, there is a need to be mindful of the Social Worker, CP Chair, or Health Visitor's need for information for a forthcoming CP conference, network meeting or legal planning meeting. With these pressures in mind, prioritisation of assessment completion and report writing means that specific information about the child and parent–child relationship can be made available in a timely way. These timescales need weekly review in the team to support individual therapists prioritise and plan their workload.

Engagement of parent–child dyads in different 'home' contexts

Additional consideration is needed when the parent and child are living with other family members, in a foster placement or a residential centre. This is because there are other relationship dynamics that impact on the relationship of the child and parent.

Adolescents/young adult parents

Often parents who are adolescents or young adults need a lot of attention and care in their own right. They can, understandably, struggle when another adult is responding more directly to their baby. The adolescent dynamic of wanting to be independent and move away from parental figures, in conflict with their feelings of needing help and dependency, is very alive. This tension and ambivalence is further complicated by the fact that the parent (young adult) now has a dependent baby who needs them to function in a mature, responsive way and needs them to prioritise their baby's needs. The example below of a mother and baby in a foster placement is an illustration of some of the themes and tensions that arise. It describes the position the therapist needed to take in relation to a parent and the foster carer.

CASE STUDY

A 3-month-old baby and her 17-year-old mother lived together in a placement with a foster carer following a pre-birth assessment. Mum had been physically assaulted and emotionally abused by her own mother (MGM) in the past. MGM and mum had been separated for most of mum's childhood. The foster carer and mum shared the same language and ethnic background.

When visited initially, the foster carer was keen for mum and herself to take part, while mum seemed overwhelmed and detached. The foster carer's inclusion in parts of the assessment seemed to help contain her own anxiety about mum and her baby, and led to her gently prompting and supporting mum to engage and consider starting the intervention. ●●●

Foster carers

Foster carers require support themselves to navigate the different and sometimes competing aspects of their role. This commonly involves finding a delicate balance between offering practical and emotional support to vulnerable young mothers while setting out the boundaries and expectations of them in their parenting role, and as a young adult in the household.

Past relationship dynamics experienced by the young parent can be quickly replicated with the foster carer, when strong emotions of rejection or blame are triggered unconsciously through their interactions. In turn, this can evoke powerful feelings in the foster carer of frustration, anxiety and rejection. These responses need time to be understood and linked to the young adult's projections, as well as commonly the foster carer's own anxiety about the welfare of both parent and baby.

There are many and varying dynamics that might need to be addressed and the therapist must negotiate pathways that provide support to both parent and child, together with the foster carer, closely liaising with the carer's supervising social worker (SSW) too. Common difficulties seen in our work included:

- young parents being superficially adult and pleasing but quickly reverting to adolescent behaviour and withdrawing from their child
- the foster carer and mother being in 'competition' for the baby's attention

- the work triggering distressing memories for the foster carer from their own life experience
- polarisation of the relationship between mother and foster carer, e.g. either too little direct help for the mother with her child, or at times too much (resulting in the mother's capacity being masked by the carer's input with the child).

Solutions are tailored to the presenting concerns but have included a combination of the following approaches in foster or residential placements. (The term foster carer may be used synonymously with residential worker where relevant. The term 'mother' is used to describe a young parent.)

- Regular feedback between the SW, SSW and SUSI worker to support the foster carer and young parent with their relationship.
- Clear, consistent communication about what expectations there are of mother in the placement in her parenting role and as an individual.
- Activity templates created for mother and child (shared with the foster carer and SW) so that goals for the parent-child relationship and progress can be observed.
- Emotional support and guidance for the foster carer, together with expectations of what kind and degree of input they offer the parent.
- Planning of general support required, e.g. boundaries around the therapy space in the home.
- Psychoeducation of babies' social-emotional development for both foster carer and parent as appropriate.
- Negotiation of the foster carer's involvement with aspects of the intervention, including advice to them regarding their responses to the child.
- Reviews to feed back progress and consider goals in the next stage.
- Support for foster carer and mother at transitions and endings.
- Consideration of signposting to services for mother's individual needs as appropriate

Communication with network

Therapeutic work can be slow to progress at times and requires a high level of liaison and clearly articulated aims for treatment, with regular reviews regarding care planning. While the direct clinical work is important, it is unlikely to succeed without the multi-agency networking and planning between appointments, especially in more complex cases.

The approach of targeting vulnerable families for assessment (used in the pilot and SUSI study), rather than using a referral system model, can be helpful with 'hard to engage' families. It addresses the difficulty for other professionals in identifying the child's needs, and families can view the offer as a standard one rather than individual or personal to them.

Key factors for the successful implementation of any service provision include leadership, joint ownership, cross boundary working, training and technical capacity (Ward, 1995, 1998; Jones, Clark, Kufeldt & Norman, 1998; Cleaver & Walker, 2004). The support at a strategic and practical level is vital so that the community multi-agency team is in a stronger position to achieve its goals. It is also more able to implement a service change that is adaptive and responsive to the network, and also clinically sensitive to a wide range of children and families with varying and competing needs.

The multi-agency agreement and support for this work in the preparation stage is central to the day to day work being integrated. Part of the joy and frustration of working in large systems is that best intentions don't always materialise, but obstacles can be surmounted with staff communicating at a grass roots level and senior staff holding a strategic overview. As with all worthwhile relationships, the essential ingredient to improving services is the hard work, commitment and dedication to understanding each other's point of view to optimise opportunities for children and families. An often unspoken but rewarding advantage of this way of working is:

- an increased understanding of each other's practice within the multi-agency groups
- individual learning about the wider system's demands
- ultimately a greater shared insight into the individual social–emotional needs of babies and very young children.

9 Training in the model

The training was well structured and organised and provided a clear insight into the work of the SUSI model. There was a real sense of commitment and expertise which translated throughout the research process and into the clinical practice.

PARENTAL MENTAL HEALTH WORKER/O.T.

The complexities and stigma surrounding parental mental health difficulties mean that parents can be particularly sensitive to advice and support, due to their feelings of guilt and shame, which results in them withdrawing from support. This training helpfully thought about ways to facilitate the more challenging conversations with parents while maintaining a supportive relationship.

PARENTAL MENTAL HEALTH SUPPORT PRACTITIONER

The training has been structured in order to deliver the core components of:

- background clinical/research literature
- the assessment and intervention processes
- inter-agency communication/liaison
- practical implementation within the clinical team and inter-agency settings in the community.

Clinical mental health work with babies, young children and their families is embedded within the community and extends across agencies and beyond traditional clinic environments. The SUSI model was designed to be deliverable in a range of environments to help with the engagement of families and to maximise their sustained involvement in the process. Alongside this, the social and family contexts for different client groups can vary a great deal, from isolated birth parents taking care of their baby single-handed with few links with community resources, to looked after children (LAC) who are part of a complex matrix involving parents/family, new primary caregivers and a wide range of professionals across multiple agencies.

Variations will be made to each training package according to the needs and service/clinical context of the team or group of practitioners being trained. Awareness of the therapists' previous mental health experience with babies and young children and the specific characteristics of their work setting will be considered, and the training programme tailored to meet the clinical and service requirements.

Whether the model is going to be delivered by a number of staff in a bespoke team or perhaps delivered by one or two members within a wider team, the work can be integrated more effectively if other staff who may not be directly involved in delivering the model have also undertaken the training. For example, if SUSI therapists were employed within an Adult or Perinatal Mental Health team, the other team members also receiving the core training would help the integration of the model. In addition, this would contribute to an understanding of how to co-ordinate work with families where the need for a parent–child intervention and parallel adult support/input is indicated. It may also be helpful to include staff who have responsibilities in cross-agency collaboration and planning at a more senior level. They would then have a strong grasp of the working practice and rationale for the introduction of a new approach and the impact of the work in a multi-agency context.

The training programme uses a combination of:

- formal teaching
- video observation tasks
- role play
- case study examples and discussion
- allocated reading
- planning for specific implementation within the team/service.

In addition, it is important to use and incorporate the existing skill base and knowledge of the team being trained to ensure their expertise is utilised within the SUSI model.

The training is divided into sections that follow the SUSI process and is delivered in a modular way. For example, after the initial training in the assessment stage, there will be follow-up sessions including consultation around specific case examples with which the team had trialled the assessment. This involves the practitioners carrying out the direct work with their supervisor's support. In the same way, after the training sessions focused on the delivery of the intervention there will be a similar approach.

An agreement needs to be made with senior staff prior to training to consider the clinical governance of the implementation of the model.

The group training will include the following key components of the SUSI clinical model and its implementation in a service setting.

1. Overview of infant and young children's developmental stages, social-emotional development and mental health presentations, parent-child attachment and relationship development for typical and maladaptive relationship patterns – this will include clinical and research background literature, health, social care and education guidance for the early years, and relevant statutory and voluntary sector reviews.
2. Training in recruitment and engagement of children and families – tailored to the specific service context and needs of the populations that the service will be available to.
3. History-taking and use of specific child and parent-child measures in the initial clinical assessment and reviews, e.g. delivery of ASQ:SE and KIPS, and administration of Denver II. While each staff member does their own e-training for KIPS, inter-rater reliability in teams requires planning.
4. Delivery of the assessment in a variety of contexts – in addition to the delivery of the clinical assessment, observations and measures, consideration should be given to:
   - ways to engage other family members where appropriate
   - clinical issues relating to the stage of the child's relationship to the caregiver and the parents/carers' mental states.
5. Report-writing – relating to the format, content and style. The report template and examples will be used as a basis for how the assessment is communicated in an accessible, written format for parents and professionals. This includes the way key aspects, components and recommendations from the initial assessment may be summarised to help facilitate engagement.
6. Liaison with and feedback of assessment to the family and network – clinical and practical issues associated with this stage of the process. This includes guidance on how to introduce the identified assessment needs and recommendations to the family and their key workers or family network in a meeting context.

7 Delivery of the intervention – training in the core components of the intervention and how they are delivered in a tailored response to the individual child and family. This will address issues relating to a range of clinical presentations in different social/family and statutory legal contexts.

8 Delivery of review assessments and the associated clinical and network liaison – training in the clinical purpose and practical aspects of engaging families for follow-up assessments along with the feedback, liaison and recommendations arising from the reviews.

9 Planning of operational systems for the specific team setting – including:
   - the establishment of inter-agency links
   - procedures for referral pathways with partner agencies
   - internal systems for tracking of referrals
   - engagement of families.

10 Review systems for case allocation – practical solutions to ensure that there is:
   - timely follow up
   - avoidance of drift
   - identification of problems and solutions for engagement and clinical work.

11 Systems for clinical record keeping and for clinical and outcomes data – advice relating to the establishment of protocols and specific databases to record quantitative and qualitative data. Guidance on how information is shared that can then be agreed within local clinical governance and inter-agency working agreements. In addition, consideration of the monitoring and evaluation of the new service offer.

12 Adaptation and use of SUSI resources to plan the creation of local psychoeducation resources – these include a range of written and visual materials developed for use with families within the engagement and intervention stages, e.g. parent information sheets, handouts on different topics and themes and individualised Activity templates.

In addition to the clinical training in the model, a one-day 'Infant Mental Health Awareness' training has been developed and delivered to a range of professionals in different community health and social care agencies. This has been extended to include follow-up learning sets for some groups to give more time to consider how workers can integrate the learning into their own practice and service approach.

10 An overview of Social-emotional Under 4s Screening and Intervention Project (SUSI)

Summary and main findings

Overview of the SUSI project

- In both a pilot project (2010–11) and follow-up feasibility study (2014–17), an infant mental health assessment and intervention model was developed and delivered in an assertive outreach approach to vulnerable populations of babies, young children and their parents/families from a community CAMHS team base in Southwark, South London. In this study, the age range included children under 4 years as we had found 4–5 year olds were generally being referred to our clinical service during the pilot project.
- Target populations included children aged 0–3 years who were: looked after; on a Child Protection Plan; children of parents engaged with mental health services.
- Key findings from the assessments included a high level of identified need across the groups, with higher than average concerns relating to the infant/child's social-emotional development, attachment and parent-child relationship, general child development and parental stress, depression and anxiety.
- The assessment informed a targeted intervention to promote the social-emotional and general development of the infant or young child and their relationships and attachment to their main caregiver(s).

- High uptake of the assessment and intervention showed its acceptability and relevance to families, and preliminary outcomes from those completing the intervention showed positive outcomes post-intervention and at 12 months follow up.
- This was not a controlled trial as the team was aware of the challenges of engaging the most vulnerable families. We also wanted to test the model which was specifically designed to address these challenges and be deliverable in the community context of multi-agency work.

Over a three year period (2014–17) a community CAMHS project team of therapists and researchers in Carelink tested the feasibility of engaging three vulnerable populations of babies, young children and their parents/families in Southwark.

The three groups of children aged 3 months to 3 years (under 4s) included:

- children who became newly looked after (LAC)
- children of parents referred to the Parental Mental Health (PMH) team
- children new to Child Protection (CP) plans.

The main aim was to provide social–emotional/mental health assessment and specific targeted interventions for babies and young children aged 0–3 years and to promote their social–emotional development and well-being, along with their attachment to their primary caregivers.

The model was developed to promote multi-agency collaboration and joint work between Mental Health, Social Care, Early Years Education and Primary Care, delivering the assessment and intervention to parents and children with colleagues in Parental Mental Health and Social Care.

We chose to run this as a feasibility study and not a controlled trial, as we were aware that the populations we were trying to engage are frequently not accessing services, partly as specialist community services are not available, and the families are in general known to be ‘hard to reach’. The study was designed to address the difficulty in engaging such stressed and traumatised families and the continuity of the staff team helped families who were anxious and stressed to agree to take part in the follow-up reviews at 6 and 12 month time-points.

Engagement of target populations

The SUSI assessment and intervention model proved to be relevant and acceptable to a diverse range of children and families with high levels of sustained engagement across a range of socio-demographic groups.

Key findings in relation to the families' participation include the following.

- 139 families were recruited in a 15-month period, each giving written informed consent.
- Of these, 88% overall completed all the baseline assessment measures.
- Of the 122 families assessed, 94% were assessed as in need of, and offered, an intervention; 86% accepted the intervention.
- 6-month review assessments were offered at 6 and 12 months, with 75% of families completing a 6-month review and 61% of families completing a 12-month review.

Socio-demographics of the consented population

- Similar numbers of girls and boys overall took part with their primary caregivers.
- Participants were from diverse ethnic backgrounds including White, Black African, Black Caribbean, Other Black, Asian, and mixed ethnicity. In total, 69% were from a Black and Minority Ethnic background.
- Overall 38% of caregivers were lone carers.
- Many of the children and families had been subject to trauma or adversity, with 41% of children having already experienced four or more 'Adverse Childhood Experiences' (ACEs).
- There was a similar rate of intervention completion across the ethnic groups.
- Nineteen mothers had had previous children removed from their care prior to the child involved in SUSI.
- The team worked hard to include fathers, resulting in between 15 to 20% involvement in the assessment and intervention phases.

Assessment process and type, and level of difficulties identified

The assessment process had core components that could be delivered to all children and families, irrespective of their current status (birth family, foster care, pre-adoptive or kinship carers) and the preferred location for the family (home, nursery, Children's Centre).

It was important there was a robust assessment that was not too burdensome for caregivers and children, many of whom were experiencing considerable pressures and distress.

Key findings from the assessments included a high level of identified need across the groups, with higher than average concerns relating to:

- the child's social-emotional development
- attachment and parent-child relationship
- general child development
- parental stress, depression and anxiety.

Outcomes of the intervention

The primary focus of the intervention was to promote the social-emotional development of the infant or young child and their relationships and attachment to their main caregiver(s).

The intervention consisted of between 10 to 15 sessions and was tailored to the individual child and their relationship, and informed by the assessment. Completion rates across the groups were high: 87% in LAC; 77% in PMH and 60% in CP.

For those families completing more than 50% of the intervention sessions (substantial therapeutic input) there were positive changes and improvements seen at the 6 month follow-up reviews in relation to the child's social-emotional development, the parent-child relationship and parent-reported levels of depression and stress.

However for families completing less than 50% of the intervention, no significant improvements were identified across any of the areas.

Importantly, the positive outcomes found at the 6 month review were also found at the 12 month follow up for all who completed more than 50% of the intervention, with the additional improvement of lower parent-reported anxiety levels at the 12 month follow-up review.

For families completing less than 50% of the intervention, no significant improvements were identified at the 12 month review.

Comparison of pre- and post-measures in the separate research groups, for everyone who was offered the intervention, regardless of how much was completed, showed the following at the 12 month review.

- The LAC group had significantly improved ASQ:SE scores and KIPS scores across the three domains (DASS was not analysed as foster carers did not complete it).
- The PMH group had significantly improved ASQ:SE mean scores, KIPS' 'promoting learning' and 'supporting confidence' scores, and parents' DASS depression, anxiety and stress scores.
- The CP group had significantly improved KIPS scores across the three domains.

Health economics evaluation

In summary, the cost of the SUSI intervention varied little between the three groups. Use and cost of other health and social care services were also similar between the three groups, apart from the higher cost of accommodation in the looked after group (as would be anticipated). There appeared to be substantial variation in health and social care cost between families, suggesting unmet need for support from health and social care services for some families.

Higher total health and social care costs per family were associated with poorer parent–child interaction and with cognitive and behavioural problems in children. Other family and child characteristics did not appear to be important predictors of cost, although the regression model explained only a small proportion of the variation, leaving room for other unobserved factors to be explored in future research (Byford & Petkova, 2017).

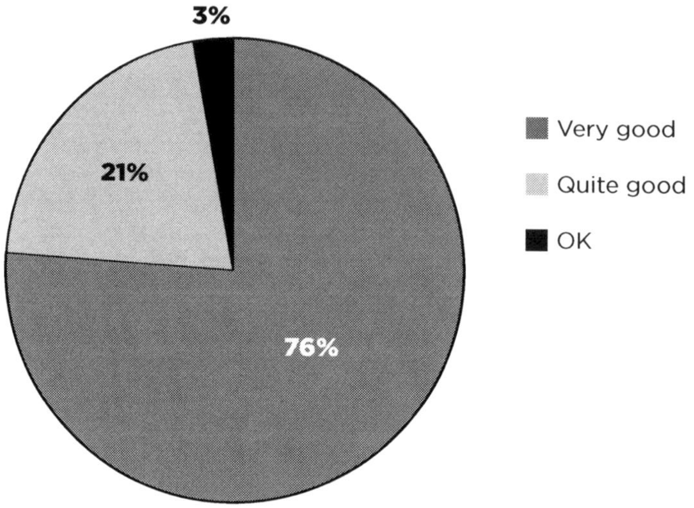

Parents/carers were asked to rate their experience of the assessment. (Note that 'Quite poor' and 'Very poor' were also options but they were not selected.)

Feedback from parents and caregivers

Parents were also asked about the usefulness of the intervention, rating this from 1–5 (with 1 being not at all useful and 5 being very useful). All parents/carers gave a rating of at least 3, with 82% rating 4 or 5. The mean rating was 4.38. Parents/carers were asked to rate how the intervention contributed to a change in the relationship with their child on a scale of 1–5 (with 1 being not at all and 5 being a great deal) – 65% gave a score of 4 or 5.

Parents also gave us detailed qualitative descriptions of what they had found to be most helpful to them.

In addition, extensive feedback was collected from social workers and health colleagues across services in interviews, focus groups and from written feedback.

Inter-agency collaboration and joint work

The model had a clear structure in order to maximise the opportunities to introduce new ways of working with Adult and Child Mental Health and community Child Health, Social Care and other agencies with key time-points set for liaison and joint work.

The SUSI team worked to engage with a wide range of professionals and family members that the primary caregiver had identified as important to them, as well as the statutory key workers who had specific responsibilities for core care planning.

In addition, the SUSI team had a significant amount of direct contact with Early Years services, including Children's Centre staff, Nursery and Foundation stage school staff, when the family's needs highlighted in the 6 and 12 month reviews were followed up.

Our colleagues in Adult Mental Health reported that the information about the child's emotional/developmental needs and the interplay between a parent's and child's needs on the developing relationship was important. It was interesting to find that the combination of assessment and feedback to the family/network was considered to be helpful in its own right.

Professionals in Children's Social Care fed back that the SUSI assessment and intervention can be delivered in complex multi-agency systems where there are multiple safeguarding issues and experience of adversity.

Dissemination and training

We have been approached by professionals in other areas of London and the UK who wish to make the case for more resources for babies, young children and families, or to establish similar services. A selection of conferences or forums that we have been invited to present at include:

- Infant Mental Health – Conception to Five conference (SLAM, London) 2019
- World Association of Infant Mental Health conference (Rome) 2018
- Looked After Children: Improving Life Chances (Manchester) 2018
- Southwark Safeguarding Executive Committee (Southwark) 2018
- Early Permanence conference (Goldsmiths, London) 2018
- Perinatal Clinical Academic group (SLAM, London) 2018
- Working with Looked After Children conference (SLAM, London) 2017
- Looking after Infant Mental Health conference (NSPCC, London) 2016
- Cornwall Infant Mental Health conference, 2016

A SUSI conference was held at the end of the project in 2017. It was attended by 150 delegates from a wide range of agencies and professional backgrounds, including Children's Social Care, Perinatal Mental Health, CAMHS, Public Health & Education, Primary Care and Parent–Infant Services.

A one-day infant mental health training workshop and a training programme for the SUSI model have been developed. The target audiences include:

- CAMHS
- Children's Social Care
- Early Help and Children's Centres
- Primary Care
- Perinatal
- Adult Mental Health.

The workshop has been delivered, along with follow-up learning sets, to groups in Early Help, Social Care and Adult Mental Health. CAMHS colleagues have been trained locally in the SUSI clinical model.

We are keen to share and discuss ideas about raising the awareness of the emotional/mental health needs of these young babies and children in community high risk groups.

We continue to explore data on the clinical presentations and profiles of babies and young children in these community populations and will disseminate findings.

References

Ainsworth, M.D.S., Blehar, M.C., Waters, E. & Wall, S. (1978). *Patterns of Attachment: A Psychological Study of the Strange Situation*. Hove, UK: Psychology Press.

Aldgate, J. & Bradley, M. (1999) *Supporting Families Through Short Term Fostering*. London: The Stationery Office.

Aldridge, H., Born, T.B., Tinson, A. & MacInnes, T. (2015). *London's Poverty Profile*. London: New Policy Institute.

All Party Parliamentary Group for Conception to Age 2 (2015) *Building Great Britons*. London: Wave Trust and PIP UK.

Anda, R.F., Felitti, V.J., Brown, D.W., Chapman, D., Dong, M., Dube S.R. ... & Giles WH. (2006) Insights into Intimate Partner Violence from the Adverse Childhood Experiences (ACE) Study. In P.R. Salber and E. Taliaferro, (Eds.) *The Physician's Guide to Intimate Partner Violence and Abuse* (pp.77–88) CA: Volcano Press.

Audit Commission (1994) *Seen But Not Heard: Co-ordinating Community Child Health and Social Services for Children in Need*. London: HMSO.

Avan, B., Richter, L.M., Ramchandani, P.G., Norris, S.A. & Stein, A. (2010). Maternal postnatal depression and children's growth and behaviour during the early years: exploring the interaction between physical and mental health. *Archives of Disease in Childhood, 95*(9).

Axford, N., Lehtonen, M., Kaoukji, D., Tobin, K. & Berry, V. (2012). Engaging parents in parenting programs: Lessons from research and practice. *Children and Youth Services, 34*, pp.2061–71.

Balbernie, R. (2016). *Infant Mental Health Services: Recognising the Importance of Relationships in the Early Years as the Foundation for Practice-Based Evidence.* Unpublished Manuscript, Parent Infant Partnership United Kingdom, Northampton, UK.

Barger, B., Rice, C., Roach, A. (2018). Socioemotional developmental surveillance in young children: monitoring and screening best identify young children that require mental health treatment. *Child and Adolescent Mental Health, 23*, pp.206–213.

Barlow, J. (2015). Parent infant psychotherapy for improving parental and infant mental health. *Cochrane Database of Systematic Reviews*.

Barlow, J., Kirkpatrick, S., Stewart-Brown, S. & Davies, H. (2005). Hard-to-Reach or Out-of-Reach? Reasons Why Women Refuse to Take Part in Early Interventions. *Children and Society, 19*, pp.199–210.

Barlow, J., Schrader-McMillan, A., Axford, N., Wrigley, Z, Sonthalia, S., Wilkinson, T. & Coad, J. (2016). Review: Attachment and attachment-related outcomes in preschool children - a review of recent evidence. *Child and Adolescent Mental Health, 21*(1), pp.11–20.

Bazalgette, L., Rahilly, T. & Trevelyan, G. (2015). *Achieving emotional wellbeing for looked after children*. London: NSPCC.

Beebe, B. & Lachmann, F.M. (2002). *Infant Research and Adult Treatment: Co-Constructing Interactions.* Hillsdale, NJ: The Analytic Press.

Bellis, M.A., Lowey, H., Leckenby, N., Hughes, K. & Harrison, D. (2014). Adverse childhood experiences: retrospective study to determine their impact on adult health behaviours and health outcomes in a UK population. *Journal of Public Health, 36*(1), pp.81–91.

Bentovim, A. (1980). Setting up the Treatment Programme. In N. Frude (Ed.), *Psychological Approaches to Child Abuse*. Guildford and Worcester: Billing & Son Ltd.

Bion, W.R. (1962b). *Learning from Experience.* London: Heinemann.

Boris, N.W., Fueyo, M. & Zeanah, C.H. (1997). The clinical assessment of attachment in children under five. *The Journal of the American Academy of Child and Adolescent Psychiatry*, 36(2), pp.291–3.

Bowlby, J. (1969). *Attachment and Loss: Volume 1. Attachment*. New York: Basic Books.

Bowlby, J. (1973). *Attachment and Loss: Volume 2: Separation*. New York: Basic Books.

Bowlby, J. (1980). *Attachment and Loss: Volume 3: Loss, Sadness and Depression*. New York: Basic Books.

Bowlby, J. (1988). *A secure base: parent-child attachment and healthy human development*. New York: Basic Books.

Brandon, M., Glaser, D., Maguire, S., McCrory, E., Lushey, C. & Ward, H. (2014). *Missed opportunities: indicators of neglect – what is ignored, why, and what can be done?* London: Department for Education, DFE-RR404, 46pp.

Brazelton, T.B. (1992). *Touchpoints: Your Child's Emotional and Behavioural Development*. New York, NY: Viking.

Brazelton, T.B., Koslowski, B. & Main, M. (1974). The origins of reciprocity: The early mother-infant interaction. In M. Lewis and L.A. Rosenblum (Eds.), *The effect of the infant on its caregiver*. New York: Wiley.

Britton, R. (1981). Re-enactment as an unwitting professional response to family dynamics. In Box, S.J., Copley, B., Magagna, J. & Moustaki, E. (Eds.), *Psychotherapy with Families: An Analytic Approach* (pp.48–58). London: Routledge.

Bronfenbrenner, U. (1979).*The Ecology of Human Development: Experiments by nature and design*. Cambridge, MA: Harvard University Press.

Bronfman, E., Parsons, E. & Lyons-Ruth, K. (1999). *Atypical Maternal Behavior Instrument for Assessment and Classification (AMBIANCE): Manual for coding disrupted affective communication. Unpublished manuscript.* Cambridge, MA: Harvard Medical School.

Buckley, H., Holt, S. & Whelan, S. (2007). Listen to me! Children's experiences of domestic violence. *Child Abuse Review, 16*, pp.296–310.

Burns, B., Phillips, S., Wagner, H., Barth, R., Kolko, D., Campbell, Y. & Landsverk, J. (2004). Mental health need and access to services by youths involved with child welfare: A national survey. *Journal of the American Academy of Child and Adolescent Psychiatry*, *43*, pp.960–970.

Byford, S. & Petkova, H. (2017). *Health Economics Evaluation*. In C. Hardy, S. Conroy & E. Murphy (Eds.), Final Grant report to Guy's and St Thomas Charity.

Cassidy, J. (1994). Emotion regulation: influences of attachment relationships. *Monographs of the Society for Research in Child Development*, *59*(2–3), pp.228–249.

Chambers, M., Saunders, A., New, B., Williams, C. & Stachurska, A. (2010). Assessment of children coming into care: Processes, pitfalls and partnerships. *Clinical Child Psychology and Psychiatry*, *15*, pp.511–527.

Cicchetti, D. & White, J. (1990). Emotion and developmental psychopathology. In N. Stein, B. Leventhal, T. Trebasso, (Eds.), *Psychological and Biological Approaches to Emotion* (pp 359–382). Hillsdale, NJ: Lawrence Erlbaum Associates.

Cleaver, H. & Walker, S. (2004). From policy to practice: the implementation of a new framework for social work assessments of children and families. *Child & Family Social Work*, *9*(1), pp.81–90.

Cleaver, H., Unell, I. & Aldgate, J. (2011). *Children's needs – Parenting capacity: The impact of parental mental illness, problem alcohol and drug use, and domestic violence on children's development. 2nd edition.* London: The Stationery Office.

Coman, W. & Devaney, J. (2011). Reflecting on Outcomes for Looked-after Children: An Ecological Perspective. *Child Care in Practice*, *17*(1), pp.37–53. http://doi.org/10.1080/13575279.2010.522976

Comfort, M. & Gordon, P. R. (2006). The Keys to Interactive Parenting Scale (KIPS): A Practical Observational Assessment of Parenting Behavior. *NHSA Dialog, 9*(1), pp.22–48.

Comfort, M., Gordon, P.R. & Unger, D.G. (2006). The Keys to Interactive Parenting Scale: A Window into Many Facets of Parenting. *Zero to Three, 26*(5), pp.37–44.

Comfort, M., Gordon, P.R. & Naples, D. (2011). KIPS: An Evidence-Based Tool for Assessing Parenting Strengths and Needs in Diverse Families. *Infants & Young Children: An Interdisciplinary Journal of Early Childhood Intervention, 24*(1), pp.56–74.

Cook, A., Spinazzola, J., Ford, J.D., Lanktree, C., Blaustein, M., Cloitre, M, ... Van der Kolk, B. (2005). Complex Trauma in Children and Adolescents. *Psychiatric Annals, 35*(5), pp.390–398.

Cowan, C.S.M., Callaghan, B.L., Kan, J.M. & Richardson, R. (2015). The lasting impact of early-life adversity on individuals and their descendants: potential mechanisms and hope for intervention. *Genes, Brain and Behavior, 15*(1), pp.155–168.

Cox, A.D., Puckering, C., Pound, A. & Mills, M. (1987). The impact of maternal depression in young children. *Journal of Child Psychology and Psychiatry, 28*(6), pp.917–928.

Crittenden, P.M. (2005). Using the CARE-Index for Screening, Intervention, and Research. Special issue: Bindungsorientierte Ansätze in der Praxis der Frühförderung 24, pp.99–106. (English on www.patcrittenden.com.)

Dabrowska, A. & Pisula, E. (2010). Parenting Stress and Coping Styles in Mothers and Fathers of Pre-School Children with Autism and Down Syndrome. *Journal of Intellectual Disability Research, 54*(3), pp.266–280.

Dallos, R. & Draper, R. (2010). *An introduction to family therapy: Systemic theory and practice*. McGraw-Hill Education (UK).

Darlington, Y. & Feeney, J. A. (2008). Collaboration between mental health and child protection services: Professionals' perceptions of best practice. *Children and Youth Services Review*, *30*(2), pp.187–198.

Darlington, Y., Feeney, J.A. & Rixon, K. (2004). Complexity, conflict and uncertainty: Issues in collaboration between child protection and mental health services. *Children and Youth Services Review, 26*, pp.1175–1192.

Darlington, Y., Feeney, J.A. & Rixon, K. (2005). Interagency collaboration between child protection and mental health services: Agency practices and perceived barriers. *Child Abuse and Neglect, 29*(10), pp.1085–1098.

Department for Education (2016). *Children Looked After: Borough*. Retrieved from: https://files.datapress.com/london/dataset/children-looked-after-borough/2016-12-01T10:44:47/children-looked-after.xls.

Department for Education and Skills (2003) *Every Child Matters (ECM)*. London: Department for Education and Skills.

Department of Health (1995) *Child Protection: Messages from Research*. London: HMSO.

Department of Health, Department for Education and Employment, Home Office (2000) *Framework for the Assessment of Children in Need and their Families*. London: The Stationery Office.

Diamond, N. & Marrone, M. (2003). *Attachment and Intersubjectivity*. Philadelphia, PA: Whurr Publishers.

Donald, M. (2001). *A Mind So Rare*. New York, NY: W.W. Norton & Co.

Early Intervention Foundation. (2016). *The Cost of Late Intervention: EIF Analysis*. London: The Early Intervention Foundation.

Emanuel, L. (2006). The contribution of organizational dynamics to the triple deprivation of looked-after children. In J. Kenrick (Ed.), *Creating New Families: Therapeutic Approaches to Fostering, Adoption and Kinship Care* (pp. 265–282). London: Karnac Books.

Erickson, E. (1968). *Identity: Youth and Crisis*. New York: W.W. Norton & Co.

Evans, G.W. (2004). The Environment of Childhood Poverty. *American Psychologist, 59*(2), pp.77–92._

Fearon, R.P., Bakermans-Kranenburg, M.J., Van Ijzendoorn, M.H., Lapsley, A.M. & Roisman, G.I. (2010). The Significance of Insecure Attachment and Disorganization in the Development of Children's Externalizing Behavior: A Meta-Analytic Study. *Child Development, 81*(2), pp.435–456.

Field, T. (2007). *The Amazing Infant.* Oxford: Blackwell.

Fonagy, P., Steele, M., Moran, G., Steele, H. & Higgitt, A. (1993). Measuring the Ghost in the Nursery: An Empirical Study of the Relation between Parents' Mental Representations of Childhood Experiences and Their Infants' Security of Attachment. *Journal of the American Psychoanalytic Association 41*(4), pp.957–989.

Fonagy P., Target, M., Steele, H. & Steele, M. (1998). *Reflective Functioning Manual. Version 5 for Application to Adult Attachment Interviews.* London: University College London.

Ford, J.D., Grasso, D., Greene, C., Levine, J., Spinazzola, J. & Van der Kolk, B. (2013). Clinical Significance of a Proposed Developmental Trauma Disorder Diagnosis: Results of an International Survey of Clinicians. *Journal of Clinical Psychiatry, 74*(8), pp.841–849.

Foreman, D. (2015). The psychiatry of children aged 0–4: advances in assessment, diagnosis and treatment. *BJ Psych Advances, 21*, pp.377–386.

Forman, D.R., O'Hara, M.W., Stuart, S., Gorman, L.L., Larsen, K.E. & Coy, K.C. (2007). Effective treatment for postpartum depression is not sufficient to improve the developing mother-child relationship. *Development and Psychopathology, 19*(2), pp.585 - 602.

Fraiberg, S. (1980). *Clinical Studies in Infant Mental Health: The First Year of Life*. New York, NY: Basic Books.

Fraiberg, S. (1982). Pathological Defenses in Infancy. *Psychoanalytic Quarterly, 51*, pp.612–635.

Fraiberg, S. (1994). *Assessment and Therapy of Disturbances in Infancy.* Northvale, NJ: Jason Aronson Inc.

Fraiberg, S., Adelson, E. & Shapiro, V. (1975). Ghosts in the Nursery: A Psychoanalytic Approach to the Problems of Impaired Infant-Mother Relationships. *Journal of the American Academy of Child Psychiatry 14*(3), pp.387–421.

Frankenburg, W.K., Dodds, J., Archer, P., Shapiro, H. & Bresnick, B. (1992). The Denver II: A Major Revision and Restandardization of the Denver Developmental Screening Test. *Pediatrics, 89*(1), pp.91–97.

Freud, S. (1923). *The Ego and the ID*. The Standard Edition of the Complete Psychological Works of Sigmund Freud, XIX (pp.1923–25): The Ego and the Id and Other Works. Vienna: W.W. Norton & Co.

Garland, C. (1998). *Understanding Trauma, a psychoanalytic approach*. London: Karnac Books.

Glascoe, F.P., Byrne, K.E., Ashford, L.G., Johnson, K.L., Chang, B. & Strickland, B. (1992). Accuracy of the Denver II in Developmental Screening. *Pediatrics, 89*(6), pp.1221–1225.

Glaser, D. (2014). The effects of child maltreatment on the developing brain. *Medico-Legal Journal, 82*(3), pp.97–111.

Goldstein, J., Freud, A. & Solnit, A. (1973). *Beyond the Best Interests of the Child.* New York: Free Press MacMillan Publishing Co.

Green, J. & Goldwyn, R. (2002). Annotation: Attachment disorganisation and psychopathology: New findings in attachment research and their potential implications for developmental psychopathology in childhood. *The Journal of Child Psychology and Psychiatry 43*(7), pp.835–846.

Green, J., Stanley, C. & Peters, S. (2007). Disorganized attachment representations and atypical parenting in young school age children with externalising disorder. *Attachment & Human Development, 9*(3), pp.207–222.

Haltigan, J.D., Madigan, S., Bronfman, E., Bailey, H.N., Borland-Kerr, C., Mills-Koonce, R. & Lyons-Ruth, K. (2019). Refining the assessment of disrupted maternal communication: Using item response models to identify central indicators of disrupted behavior. *Development and Psychopathology, 31*(1), pp.261–277.

Hardy, C. (2001). Infants and Young Children. In L. Lougher (Ed.), *Occupational Therapy for Child and Adolescent Mental Health* (pp.113–131). London: Churchill Livingstone.

Hardy, C. & Murphy, E., (2013) Social-emotional screening and intervention for 0–4 year old children entering care. In M. Tarren-Sweeney & A. Vetere (Eds.), *Mental Health Services for Vulnerable Children and Young People* (pp.102–116). London: Routledge.

Hardy, C., Hackett, E., Murphy, E., Cooper, B., Ford, T. & Conroy, S. (2015). Mental health screening and early intervention: Clinical research study for under 5-year-old Children in Care in an inner London borough. *Clinical Child Psychology and Psychiatry 20*(2), pp.261–275.

Hardy, C. & Murphy, E. (2018). Workshop WS82 Social-emotional assessment and intervention for 0–3s in high risk populations (SUSI study). 16th World Congress. *Infant Mental Health Journal*, Supplement to Vol. 39.

Health and Social Care Committee. 'First 1000 days of life inquiry'. (2018) UK Parliamentary website. Retrieved from https://www.parliament.uk/business/committees/committees-a-z/commons-select/health-and-social-care-committee/inquiries/parliament-2017/first-1000-days-life-inquiry-17-19/

Heimann, P. (1950). On counter-transference. *The International Journal of Psychoanalysis, 31*, pp.81–84.

Henry, J.D. & Crawford, J.R., (2005). The short-form version of the Depression Anxiety Stress Scales (DASS-21): Construct validity and normative data in a large non-clinical sample. *British Journal of Clinical Psychology, 44*(2), pp.227–239.

Hertzman, C. & Boyce, T. (2010). How Experience Gets Under the Skin to Create Gradients in Developmental Health. *Annual Review of Public Health, 31*, pp.329–347.

Hetherington, R., Baistrow, K., Katz, I., Mesie, J. & Trowell, J. (2002). *The welfare of children with mentally ill parents: Learning from inter-country comparisons*. Chichester: John Wiley & Sons.

Hindle, D. & Shulman, G. (2008). *The Emotional Experience of Adoption: A psychoanalytic perspective.* Oxford: Routledge.

Hopkins, J. (1992). Infant-Parent Psychotherapy. *Journal of Child Psychotherapy, 18*, 5–17.

Hudson, B. (2002). Interprofessionality in health and social care: The Achilles' heel of partnership? *Journal of Interprofessional Care, 16*(1), pp.7–17.

Johnson, L.J., Zorn, D., Kai Yung Tam, B., Lamontage, M. & Johnson, S. A. (2003). Stakeholders' views of factors that impact successful interagency collaboration. *Exceptional Children, 69*(2), pp.195–209.

Jones, H., Clark, R., Kufeldt, K. & Norman, M. (1998) Looking After Children: assessing outcomes in child care: the experience of implementation. *Children and Society*, 12**,** pp.212–222.

Jowett, S., Karatzias, T., Shevlin, M. & Albert, I. (2020). Differentiating Symptom Profiles of ICD-11 PTSD, Complex PTSD, and Borderline Personality Disorder: A Latent Class Analysis in a Multiply Traumatized Sample. *Personality Disorders*, 11 (1), pp.36–45.

Kavanagh, D.J., Piatkowska, O., Clark, D., O'halloran, P., Manicavasagar, V., Rosen, A. & Tennant, C. (1993). Application of Cognitive-Behavioural Family Intervention for Schizophrenia in Multidisciplinary Teams: What Can the Matter Be? *Australian Psychologist, 28*(3), pp.181–188.

Klein, M. (1928). Early stages of the Oedipus conflict. *International Journal of psychoanalysis, 9*, pp.169–180.

Klein, M. (1959). Our Adult World and its Roots. In M. Klein, *Envy and Gratitude: and Other Works*. London: Vintage.

Langner, T.S. & Michael, S.T. (1963). *Life stress and mental health: II. The midtown Manhattan study* (Vol. 2). Oxford: Free Press Glencoe.

Lieberman, A.F. & Pawl, J.H. (1990). Disorders of Attachment and Secure Base Behaviour in the Second Year of Life: Conceptual Issues and Clinical Intervention. In M.T. Greenberg, D. Cicchetti & E.M. Cummings (Eds.), *Attachment in the Preschool Years: Theory, Research and Intervention* (pp.375–396). Chicago, IL: University of Chicago Press.

Lieberman, A.F. & Van Horn, P. (2008). *Psychotherapy with Infants and Young Children: Repairing the Effects of Stress and Trauma on Early Attachment.* New York, NY: The Guilford Press.

Lomanowska, A., Boivin, M., Hertzman, C. & Fleming, A.S. (2015). Parenting Begets Parenting: A Neurobiological Perspective on Early Adversity and the Transmission of Parenting Styles Across Generations. *Neuroscience, 342*, pp.120–139.

Lovibond, S.H. Lovibond, P.F. (1995) *Manual for the depression anxiety stress scales*. Sydney Psychology Foundation.

Lyons-Ruth, K. (2003). Dissociation and the Parent–Infant Dialogue: A Longitudinal Perspective from Attachment Research. *Journal of the American Psychoanalytic Association, 51*(1), pp.883–911.

Lyons-Ruth, K. (2008). Contributions of the Mother–Infant Relationship to Dissociative, Borderline, and Conduct Symptoms in Young Adulthood. *Infant Mental Health Journal 29*(3), pp.203–218.

Lyons-Ruth, K., Bronfman, E. & Parsons, E. (1999). Maternal frightened, frightening, or atypical behavior and disorganized infant attachment patterns. *Monographs of the Society for Research in Child Development*, pp.67–96.

Mahler, M.S., Pine, F. & Bergman, A. (1975) *The Psychological Birth of the Human Infant.* New York: Basic Books.

Main, M. (2000). The Organized Categories of Infant, Child, and Adult Attachment: Flexible Vs. Inflexible Attention Under Attachment-Related Stress. *Journal of American Psychoanalytic Association, 48*, pp.1055–1096.

Main, M. & Solomon, J. (1986). Discovery of an insecure–disorganized/disoriented attachment pattern. In T. B. Brazelton & M. W. Yogman (Eds.), *Affective development in infancy* (pp. 95–124). Westport, CT, US: Ablex Publishing.

McClosky, L., Figueredo, A. & Koss, P. (1995) The effects of systemic family violence on children's mental health. *Child Development*, *66*, pp.1239–1261.

McCrory, E., De Brito,S.A. & Viding, E. (2010). Research Review: The neurobiology and genetics of maltreatment and adversity. *Journal of Child Psychology and Psychiatry, 51*(10), pp.1079–1095.

McCrory, E.J., Gerin, M.I. & Viding, E. (2017). Annual research review: childhood maltreatment, latent vulnerability and the shift to preventative psychiatry – the contribution of functional brain imaging. *Journal of Child Psychology and Psychiatry*, *58*(4), pp.338–357.

McMahon, C.A. & Meins, E. (2012). Mind-mindedness, parenting stress, and emotional availability in mothers of pre-schoolers. *Early Childhood Research Quarterly 27*(1), pp.245–252.

Meins, E. (1998) The effects of security attachment and material attribution of meaning on children's linguistic acquisitional style. *Infant Behavior and Development, 21*(2), pp.237–252.

Moriarty, J., Baginsky, W., Gorin, S., Baginsky, M. & Manthorpe, J. (2016). *Mapping mental health services for looked after children in London aged 0–5 years*. London: The Policy Institute, Kings College London.

Murray, L. (2005). *The Social Baby: Understanding Babies' Communication from Birth*. Richmond: CP Publishing.

Murray, L. (2014). *The psychology of babies: how relationships support development from birth to two*. UK: Hachette.

Murray, L., Cooper, P., Wilson, A. & Romani, H. (2003). Controlled trial of the short- and long-term effect of psychological treatment of post-partum depression: 2. Impact on the mother–child relationship and child outcome. *The British Journal of Psychiatry 182* (5), pp.420 – 427.

Murray, L., De Pascalis, L., Bozicevic, L., Hawkins, L., Sclafani, V. & Ferrari, P. F. (2016). The functional architecture of mother-infant communication, and the development of infant social expressiveness in the first two months. *Scientific Reports, 6*, pp.1–9.

Music, G. (2011). *Nurturing Natures: Attachment and Children's Emotional, Sociocultural and Brain Development.* Hove, UK: Psychology Press.

Music, G. (2017). *Growing an Emotional Brain*. Retrieved from https://www.youtube.com/watch?v=hVN0YzBVAKQ.

Myers, J.E.B., Berliner, L., Briere, J., Hendrix, C.T., Jenny, C. & Reid, T.A. (Eds.). (2002). *The APSAC handbook on child maltreatment* (2nd ed.). Sage Publications, Inc.

NICE: National Institute for Health and Care Excellence (2012). Social and emotional wellbeing: early years. Retrieved from: https://www.nice.org.uk/guidance/ph40

NICE: National Institute for Health and Clinical Excellence and Social Care Institute for Excellence (2010). *Looked-after children and young people: Promoting the quality of life of looked after children and young people*. London, UK: NICE (PH28).

NICE: National Institute for Health and Care Excellence, (2014). *Antenatal and postnatal mental health: clinical management and service guidance*. NICE (CG192). Updated Feb 2020.

NICE: National Institute for Health and Care Excellence, (2017). *Child Abuse and Neglect.* NICE Guideline (NG76).

NSPCC (2016). *Looking After Infant Mental Health: Our Case for Change: A Summary of Research Evidence*. London: NSPCC.

O'Keefe, M. (1995) Predictors of child abuse in maritally violent families. *Journal of Interpersonal Violence*, *10*, 3–25.

Olds, D.L., Robinson, J., O'Brien, R., Luckey, D.W., Pettitt, L.M., Henderson, C.R., ... & Talmi, A. (2002). Home visiting by paraprofessionals and by nurses: a randomized, controlled trial. *Pediatrics, 110*(3), pp.486–496.

Piek, J.P., Barrett, N.C., Smith, L.M., Rigoli, D. & Gasson, N. (2010) Do motor skills in infancy and early childhood predict anxious and depressive symptomatology at school age? *Human Movement Science, 29*(5), pp.777–786.

Piontelli, A. (1992). *From Fetus to Child: Observational and Psychoanalytical Study*. London: Routledge.

PIP UK (2019) *Rare jewels. Specialised parent–infant relationship teams in the UK*. Parent Infant Partnership, UK. Retrieved from: https://parentinfantfoundation.org.uk/our-work/campaigning/rare-jewels/.

Prior, V. & Glaser, D. (2006). *Understanding Attachment and Attachment Disorders: Theory, Evidence and Practice.* London: Jessica Kingsley Publishers.

Ramsdal, G., Bergvik, S. & Wynn, R. (2015). Parent–child attachment, academic performance and the process of high-school drop-out: a narrative review. *Attachment & Human Development, 17*(5), pp.522–545.

Raphael-Leff, J. (1991). *Psychological Processes of Childbearing*. London: Chapman and Hall.

Schore, A.N. (2001). Effects of secure attachment on right brain development. *Infant Mental Health Journal, 22*, pp.7–66.

Scott, D. (2010). Working within and between organisation. In F. Arney & D. Scott (Eds.), *Working with Vulnerable families: A partnership approach*. Cambridge, UK: Cambridge University Press.

Segal, H. (1964). *Introduction to the work of Melanie Klein*. London: Heinemann.

Slade, A. (2005). Parental reflective functioning: an introduction. *Attachment & Human Development*, 7(3), pp.269-281.

Slade, A., Grienenberger, J., Bernbach, E. Levy, D. & Locker, A. (2005). Maternal reflective functioning, attachment, and the transmission gap: A preliminary study. *Attachment & Human Development, 7*(3), pp.283–298.

Social Care Institute for Excellence. (2017) Improving mental health support for our children and young people. Expert Working Group report. Retrieved from https://www.scie.org.uk/children/care/mental-health/report.

Squires, J., Bricker, D. & Twombly, E. (2003). *The ASQ:SE user's guide*. Maryland: Paul H. Brooks Publishing Co.

Squires, J., Bricker, D. & Twombly, E. (2015). *Ages & Stages Questionnaires: Social–emotional (ASQ:SE-2™) A Parent-Completed Child Monitoring System for Social–Emotional Behaviours.* Maryland: Paul H. Brooks Publishing Co.

Sroufe, L.A. (2005). Attachment and development: A prospective, longitudinal study from birth to adulthood. *Attachment & Human Development, 7*(4), pp.349–367. http://doi.org/10.1080/14616730500365928.

Stanley, N., Penhale, B., Riordan, D., Barbour, R.S. & Holden, S. (2003). Working on the interface: Identifying professional responses to families with mental health and child-care needs. *Health and Social Care in the Community, 11*(3), pp.208–218.

Steele, H. & Siever, L. (2010). An Attachment Perspective on Borderline Personality Disorder: Advances in Gene-Environment Considerations. *Current Psychiatry Reports, 12*(1), pp.61–67.

Stern, D.N. (1985). *The Interpersonal World of the Infant: A View from Psychoanalysis and Developmental Psychology*. New York, NY: Basic Books.

Stern, D.N. (1995). *The Motherhood Constellation: A Unified View of Parent–Infant Psychotherapy.* New York, NY: Basic Books.

Stern, D.N. (2002). *The First Relationship: Infant and Mother.* Cambridge, MA: Harvard University Press.

Stovall-McClough, K.C. & Dozier, M. (2004). Forming attachments in foster care: Infant attachment behaviors during the first 2 months of placement. *Development and Psychopathology, 16*(2), pp.253–271.

Teicher, M.H. & Samson J.A. (2016). Annual Research Review: Enduring neurobiological effects of childhood abuse and neglect. *Journal of Child Psychology and Psychiatry, 57*(3), pp.241–266.

The National Scientific Council on the Developing Child. (2014). *Excessive Stress Disrupts the Architecture of the Developing Brain.* Cambridge, MA: Harvard.

Trauma Centre at Justice Resource Institute. (2012). *Developmental Trauma Disorder: Field Trial Phase III*. Retrieved from: http://www.traumacenter.org/research/DTD_Field_Trial.php.

Trevarthen, C. & Aitken, K.J. (2001). Infant Intersubjectivity: Research, Theory, and Clinical Applications. *The Journal of Child Psychology and Psychiatry, 42*(1), pp.3–48.

Tronick, E.Z. (1989). Emotions and Emotional Communication in Infants. *American Psychologist, 44*(2), pp.112–119.

Van der Kolk, B.A. (2005). Developmental Trauma Disorder: Toward a rational diagnosis for children with complex trauma histories. *Psychiatric Annals, 35*(5), pp.401–408.

Van der Kolk, B.A. (2015). *The body keeps the score: Brain, mind, and body in the healing of trauma*. London: Penguin Books.

Van der Kolk, B.A., Pynoos, R.S., Cicchetti, D., Cloitre, M., D'Andrea, W., Ford, J.D., ... Teicher, M. (2009). *Proposal to Include a Developmental Trauma Disorder Diagnosis for Children and Adolescents in DSM-V.* Retrieved from: http://www.traumacenter.org/announcements/DTD_NCTSN_official_submission_to_DSM_V_Final_Version.pdf

Van Ijzendoorn, M.H., Schuengel, C. & Bakermans-Kranenburg, M.J. (1999). Disorganized attachment in early childhood: Meta-analysis of precursors, concomitants, and sequelae. *Development and Psychopathology, 11*(2), pp.225–250.

Ward, H. (1995). Research messages for implementation. In H. Ward (Ed.), *Looking After Children: Research into Practice* (pp. 109–128). London: HMSO.

Ward, H. (1998) Using a child development model to assess the outcomes of social work interventions with families. *Children and Society*, *12*(3), pp.202–211.

Winnicott, D.W. (1960). The Theory of Parent–Infant Relationship. *International Journal of Psychoanalysis*, *41*, pp.585–595.

World Health Organization (2019). International statistical classification of diseases and related health problems (11th ed.). https://icd.who.int/.

Zeanah, C.H., Berlin, L.J. & Boris, N.W. (2011). Practitioner Review: Clinical applications of attachment theory and research for infants and young children. *The Journal of Child Psychology and Psychiatry 52*(8), pp.819–833.

Zero to Three. (2005). *Diagnostic classification of mental health and developmental disorders of infancy and early childhood: Revised edition* (DC: 0–3R). Washington, DC: Zero To Three Press.

Zero to Three. (2016). *Diagnostic classification of mental health and developmental disorders of infancy and early childhood: Revised edition* (DC: 0–5). Washington, DC: Zero To Three Press.

Notes

Notes

Notes